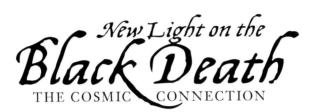

New Light on the

Black Death

THE COSMIC CONNECTION

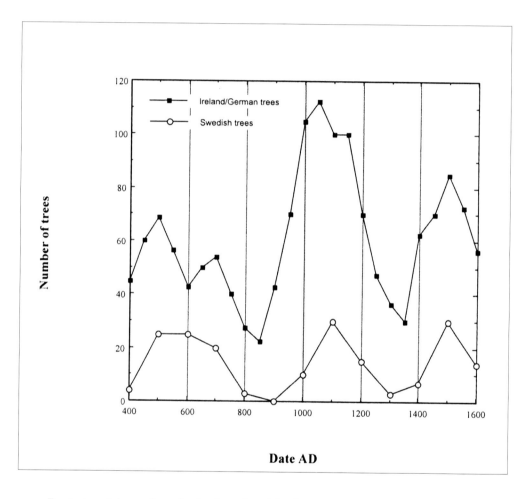

Frontispiece: A lesson from dendrochronology. The figure shows the number of Irish and German oaks through time compared with the number of pines from Swedish lakes. It is always assumed that the number of oaks found in buildings and on archaeological sites is influenced mainly by human activity. However, the number of pines in Swedish lakes is an entirely natural phenomenon; not influenced by humans. QED the oak replication is actually a reflection of the influence of the environment on human activity and it is the environment that is driving the system. *German and Swedish data courtesy of Hubert Leuschner and Bjorn Gunnarson respectively*

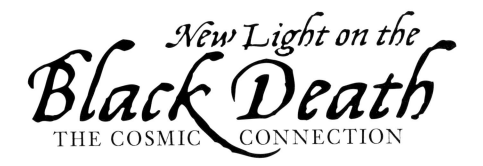

New Light on the Black Death
THE COSMIC CONNECTION

MIKE BAILLIE

TEMPUS

Dedicated to Fred Hoyle and Chandra Wickramasinghe who got closer to the cause of the Black Death than anyone since the fourteenth century

First published 2006

Tempus Publishing Limited
The Mill, Brimscombe Port,
Stroud, Gloucestershire, GL5 2QG
www.tempus-publishing.com

British Library Cataloguing in Publication Data.
A catalogue record for this book is available from the British Library.

ISBN 0 7524 3598 1

Typesetting and origination by Tempus Publishing Limited
Printed in Great Britain

CONTENTS

PREFACE

This book was written because in the academic year 2003-4 I was granted sabbatical leave from Queen's University, Belfast. When such leave is being applied for it is normal to map out the objectives – what can the university expect in return for the privilege of a year free to undertake research? In the circumstances, and egged on by just a hint of bravado, and an offer from Peter Kemmis Betty at Tempus, I said I was going to write *two* books. What happened was marginally different. With a co-author, Patrick McCafferty, I managed to finish one book entitled *The Celtic Gods: comets in Irish mythology*. The other, this book, only got off the ground during that year. It was to take another year, and more, in the writing.

All of this gave me the chance to develop what had only been a loose idea about a book on the Black Death. I think it is fair to say that this is a book which is not quite like any other on the topic. I'm not going to concentrate on the normal historical aspects of the disease and its spread, as most books on the subject feel obliged to do. This is because I'm not an historian. Instead, as a dendrochronologist and a palaeoecologist (i.e. someone interested in chronology and past environmental change), I try to see what story can be conjured from the wide-ranging scientific evidence relating to any given period; in this case the fourteenth century. So this book is an attempt to pull together a picture of the environmental happenings across the fourteenth century that can act as a backdrop for the plague, whatever it was, that arrived into Europe in 1348.

Some of the content of the book could be described as 'educated speculation'. However this speculation is rooted in a host of scientific evidence, from a variety of fields, most of which will probably be unfamiliar to researchers in the broad field of historical research. In this I have been helped enormously by the generosity of colleagues in the fields of dendrochronology (tree-ring studies), ice cores, pollen, tephra, radiocarbon and environmental change.

To explain: in the 1990s, I found myself in the privileged position of having access to more long tree-ring chronologies that just about anyone else on the planet. Colleagues around the world, with almost unbelievable generosity, were happy to provide me with their data. These tree-ring chronologies, all precisely dated, covered a wide geographical spread, and allowed me, for the first time, to attempt to gauge what trees were recording globally across this most interesting century. From the dendrochronological community I would like to thank particularly Keith Briffa, Ed Cook, Deiter Eckstein, Don Graybill, Cathy Groves, Hakan Grudd, Peter Kuniholm, Antonio Lara, Chung Lemin, Hubert Leuschner, Stepan Shiyatov, Ian Tyers, Eugene Vaganov and Ricardo Villalba. The staff at the Laboratory for Tree-Ring Research, University of Arizona, Tucson, have been helpful as always in dealing with requests for data or information. For help with information on dated tephra layers I wish to thank Valerie Hall and Jon Pilcher; for inter-hemispheric radiocarbon calibration information Alan Hogg, Gerry McCormac and Paula Reimer, and for information on sea-surface temperatures Alistair Dawson. From the ice-core community I need to thank Henri Clausen for sharing information on the European GRIP ice-core analyses, and Kendrick Taylor and Paul Mayewski for providing the GISP2 chemistry record. All the data from the ice cores was obtained from *The Greenland Summit Ice Cores CD-ROM. 1997*, available from the National Snow and Ice Data Centre, University of Colorado at Boulder, and the World Data Centre-A for Paleoclimatology, National Geophysical Data Centre, Boulder, Colorado. I would stress that what I have done with the GISP2 record is entirely my idea, and my responsibility, though I trust the logic of my re-dating of a section of the GISP2 ice core will be accepted. I would also like to thank Eric Wolff for his help in preventing a compromising error with respect to an anomaly in the twelfth century BC in the Antarctic, DomeC, ice core. I would like to thank Jon Pilcher, Patrick McCafferty and Peter Kemmis Betty for reading drafts of the text and offering constructive suggestions and Libby Mulqueeny for assistance with some of the drawings. If I have omitted anyone through oversight I hope they will understand.

Given the nature of the evidence-based story that emerges in the course of this book, hopefully it will read more like a Dan Brown *Da Vinci Code* than a dry textbook. The sheer variety of information, coupled with the real puzzle that is the environmental past, means that the interested reader will be led down some strange paths. It is my firm belief that the environment had more of a hand in the plague known as the Black Death than is generally realized. The 'Grail' in this case is the understanding of what environmental trigger *caused* the plague; a plague that killed about one third of Europe's population. By the end it will be clear that, the 'secret of the environmental Grail' is close, but it is not yet completely to hand. It is proving almost as elusive in this book as was the quest in the *Code* (almost as elusive, but not quite; because I think we are getting there). Hopefully, with this book, at least some of the groundwork has now been laid for the eventual full integration of the environment into the history of the fourteenth century.

INTRODUCTION

It is important to know where I am coming from in attempting to put this book together. Through tree-rings, and the environmental events highlighted by them, I have become an environmental catastrophist. I did not start out as one, but in attempting to get a handle on some key environmental events in the last five millennia I have been driven to recognise that human populations have been subjected to rather more catastrophic events than is normally realized. When precisely dated tree-ring events coincide in time with major cultural changes, or dynastic changes, or famines, or plagues – *as they undoubtedly do* – then it is beholden on us to attempt to understand what caused the environmental events. However, what I had never suspected, until I tried to understand what was happening around key environmental events such as those at 2350 BC, 1150 BC or AD 540, was that *dated* myths and metaphors can provide real and useful information. In order to understand past environmental events properly it is important to know how to handle such information. This is where a multi-disciplinary approach is helpful.

Over recent years scholars have been driven more and more into specialism. There is so much literature in every field that it is well-nigh impossible for researchers to read outside their own subject areas. Thus relatively few people in, say, economic history or historical geography will know how much tree-ring, or radiocarbon, or ice-core information is available. Almost none will know how to interpret what is normally regarded as marginal literature on a subject like mythology. In fact, there is a lot of relevant information out there, but it's in specialist journals, unlikely to be read by a wider audience. My feeling is that interdisciplinary study will have to make a comeback if we are ever to gain a true picture of what affected human populations, even in relatively recent times.

In the nineteenth century the German historian J.F.C. Hecker produced a list of terrible, bizarre, happenings in the Orient in the run up to the Black Death. His start date was AD 1333. He describes peculiar earthquakes lasting for days, violent torrents of rain, tectonic movements, millions of deaths, uncommon atmospheric phenomena, water springing from rocks, destructive deluges and unheard-of inundations and:

> a fiery meteor, which descended on the earth far in the East … destroyed everything within a circumference of more than a hundred leagues, infecting the air far and wide.

> …We find notice of an unexampled earthquake, which on the twenty fifth of January 1348, shook Greece, Italy, and the neighbouring countries.

To which he adds 'Great and extraordinary meteors appeared in many places'.[1] That is the gist of what he says. But it is interesting to see the *tone* of his comments on this list. Basically, looking at the list he was drawing up, he said that a great natural upheaval shook the earth for 26 years following 1333. In his view, the air was affected by this upheaval, in fact, as he put it:

> This disease was a consequence of violent commotions in the earth's organism – if any disease of cosmical origin can be so considered.

So Hecker was pretty sure that the Black Death was part of a package, and he felt it would be unwise to pick bits of the story in trying to understand 'the causes of a cosmical commotion, which has never recurred to an equal extent'. This present book is going to look at a range of data – now available to the scientific community – that sits surprisingly comfortably with Hecker's views. I'm going to show that there does seem to have been a 'violent commotion of the earth's organism', quite possibly starting in 1333, but focusing uncomfortably on January 1348.

Another writer who sets the correct tone for study of the Black Death is Jon Arrizabalaga.[2] I was introduced to Arrizabalaga's work by Ben Dodds at a time when I was trying to envisage the best way to present the various strands of information that I think the reader needs in order to fully understand the problem of the fourteenth century. Arrizabalaga makes the significant point that we should not view the plague of the mid-fourteenth century from a modern laboratory standpoint – a position wherein lies the tendency to 'tell' the disease, and the people who experienced it, how it/they should have behaved (had it been a modern disease and had they owned a modern treatise on plague); rather, we need to try to see the disease, and the conditions surrounding it's arrival, from a medieval perspective. Hopefully, the scientific information now available, concerning the environment of the fourteenth century, is sufficiently independent of modern medical perceptions to allow an independent view to be developed.

Circumstances, however, allow the situation to be even better than this. Because the long tree-ring chronologies have allowed the viewing of a series of environmental catastrophes in the more distant past – for example, in the twenty-fourth, twelfth and third centuries BC, and in the sixth century AD – the possibility now exists to effectively view the fourteenth century from the past. The importance of this approach is that it allows prior experience of 'patchy historical recording of catastrophic events' – often in myth and unsupported individual accounts – to be applied to the almost equally patchy record of the years running up to 1350. It is possible to demonstrate how quite accurate accounts of ancient happenings can be conjured from *dated* myth and metaphor. This is possible when we have access to well-dated scientific records of environmental happenings, such as those provided by dendrochronology and ice-core research, to allow proper interpretation of the surviving records. To generalize Arrizabalaga's idea, it can be suggested that the correct perspective for the Black Death is to view it as the *last* of a list of catastrophes that have taken place over the last few millennia. In that way we are forced to look afresh at the information that has been systematically marginalized by modern historical scholarship.

As will become clear in the text, in line with Arrizabalaga's suggestion, it is not possible to understand the Black Death without a particular understanding of the prequel plague which struck Europe around AD 540, during the reign of the Byzantine emperor Justinian. The Justinian plague seems to be a much better model for the fourteenth-century Black Death than any localized late nineteenth-century outbreak of bubonic plague. For those not familiar with any of these issues what follows is a short section on the conventional wisdom with respect to the Black Death. Hopefully it contains enough information to get the beginner started.

THE CONVENTIONAL WISDOM AND SOME OF ITS PROBLEMS

This book is not much concerned with the conventional wisdom on the nature of the Black Death. The aim is to throw some new light on the *other* things that were going on at the time of the great fourteenth-century pandemic. However, it is probably necessary to make some sort of statement to set the scene for the discussion. Here is a very loose paraphrase of what has generally been taught about the fourteenth-century plague. The Black Death of 1347 was believed to be the third great outbreak of bubonic plague; a plague that is traditionally spread by rats and fleas. The previous instances were the Plague of Athens in 430 BC and the plague at the time of Justinian which arrived into Constantinople in AD 542. The Plague of Athens was described by Thucydides, while the Justinian plague was described by Procopius, among others. One key issue in the conventional story is that the symptoms of the plague included buboes in the arm-pit or groin of the victims who generally died within a few days of infection. These symptoms have been repeated endlessly as a defining characteristic of bubonic plague.

The plague is supposed to have originated in Central Asia, or somewhere in Africa, where plague is endemic in some rodent populations. It is assumed that some environmental stimulus caused infected rodents to leave their normal habitats and infect rat populations, and ultimately human populations, in areas where there was no natural immunity. The mechanism of transfer is believed to have been infected fleas leaving the bodies of dead rats and moving to human hosts who were in turn infected by the feeding fleas. It is believed that trade routes brought the disease to the Black Sea region and from there to the central Mediterranean by late 1347. It was then introduced into Europe through northern Italy and southern France. It immediately started killing people in large numbers, spreading overland at about 1.5km per day. Between January and the summer to autumn of 1348 it had spread as far as the British Isles, and by 1350 to Scandinavia and eventually even Iceland. The spread seems to have curled up through France, across Belgium into Germany and on into central, southern Europe. This first wave burned itself out by 1351, though there was a second wave in 1361.

It is generally believed that the plague hit an already weakened population in Europe. The flowering of the thirteenth century had gone into reverse in the early fourteenth century with worsening climatic conditions, including the devastatingly wet years of 1315-7 with widespread crop failures and famine. So the Black Death, with an unusually (indeed abnormally) high death rate, made more sense if it was striking a population weakened by famine.

If that was roughly the conventional wisdom, the last 20 years have seen increasing questioning of that wisdom. At its most basic, the problem is with those rats and fleas. For the conventional wisdom to work there have to be hosts of infected rats and they have to be moving at alarming speed – you would almost have to imagine infected rats scuttling ever onward (mostly northward) delivering, as they died, their loads of infected fleas. The snags with this scenario are legion. For example, there are no descriptions of dead rats lying everywhere (this is explained by suggesting that either the rats were indoors, or people were so used to dead rats that they were not worth mentioning; though if they were indoors how did they travel so fast?). It did not seem to matter whether you were a rural shepherd or cleric or a town dweller, both were infected. Yet strangely with this very infectious disease some cities across Europe were spared. Moreover, these rats must have been happy to move to cool northern areas even though bubonic plague is a disease that requires relatively warm temperatures. Then, when there are water barriers, these rats board ships to keep the momentum going. To these quibbles we can add what contemporary writers recorded. What people at the time made note of was the *remarkable* kill rate. They had never heard of such high mortalities, up to 30 per cent and even 50 per cent. They also referred to the 'corruption of the atmosphere' which was what some people thought the plague actually was.

Issues such as these forced some historians to move a little from the rats/fleas scenario. In order to get away from the peculiarity of the fourteenth-century rats/fleas, it was decided that most of the deaths must have been due to the pneumonic form of the disease that could be transmitted from person to person. The snag with this idea is that pneumonic plague is hard to identify in contemporary descriptions. Basically doubts were starting to accumulate with the conventional bubonic plague

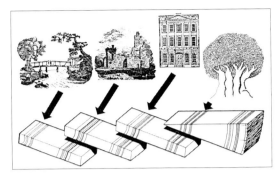

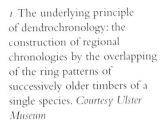

1 The underlying principle of dendrochronology: the construction of regional chronologies by the overlapping of the ring patterns of successively older timbers of a single species. *Courtesy Ulster Museum*

story. This was when new hypotheses began to be promoted. In 1984 Graham Twigg tackled the issue head on and suggested that bubonic plague made no sense – killing people in the winter in northern Europe – the killer had to be something else, possibly something like anthrax.[3] Around the same time, Fred Hoyle and Chandra Wickramasinghe went one further and suggested that the spread bore more resemblance to something spreading through the air. Indeed they went so far as to suggest that the disease actually entered the atmosphere from space, descending at differing rates and thus spreading over a few years (*Appendix 1*).[4]

More recently, Cohn has pointed out that the kill rates reported in the fourteenth century were completely different from those observed around 1900 in India and China, where bubonic plague would kill only about 3 per cent of a population, not 30 per cent or more.[5] Perhaps the following anecdote, based on Cohn's work, will sum up the problem of the Black Death. Apparently doctors treating people with bubonic plague, around 1900, observed that it was quite hard to spread the infection. Infected people in hospitals were visited by relatives who did not get sick, most doctors and nurses did not get the disease. Yet some of these doctors were quite capable of writing that the disease was 'highly contagious'. Why would they observe one thing and record the opposite? The answer seems to lie in what they were *taught* as medical students, namely that the Black Death *was* bubonic plague and it *was* highly contagious. So ingrained was this prejudice, that experienced medical personnel were capable of denying what they were seeing with their own eyes. Cohn also points out that people's reaction to the plague's first arrival in 1348 was one of hopelessness in the face of something 'new to world history', indeed something sent by God. The widespread reaction was that there was no remedy. Later, after 1350, this hopelessness changed to a situation where more emphasis was placed on 'remedies, cures and preventive measures'.[6]

If you wanted a good reason to doubt that the Black Death was bubonic plague, these four authors provide plenty of ammunition. But, and here is the rub, if the Black Death was not bubonic plague, then, we need to know what it was! Given that it is widely accepted as having killed one third of Europe's population, it is alarming, to say the least, that we may not know its identity. If some *unknown* agent could kill one third of Europe's population a mere six centuries ago, presumably it could arrive again and do the same thing tomorrow! By the end of this book readers will have further reasons for doubting the conventional wisdom.

However, just in case the reader gets the feeling from this brief background that all scholars are moving away from bubonic plague, it is worth commenting on one recent book. Benedictow[7] does not believe that there was any significant airborne component; he believes in an advancing 'army' which was the Black Death 'riding triumphantly and invisibly in the bodies of rodents or their consort of fleas'. The terminology is consistently military with the 'forces' of the 'advancing army' 'marching' through 'campaign' to 'invasion' and 'conquest'. So Benedictow is in no doubt about the rat/flea transmission vector. He even at one point elaborates:

> The Black Death's strategic genius made also another masterstroke that greatly increased the pace of its conquest of the Iberian Peninsula. Shortly after its multiple invasions of important urban centres along the coast of the Kingdom of Aragon, it performed a remarkable metastatic leap and arrived triumphantly in the town of Santiago de Compostela in the very opposite, north-westernmost corner of the Iberian Peninsula.[8]

It is easy to see why people might start to have doubts about the rat/flea hypothesis when they see it imbued not only with malicious intent, but, indeed, with the ability to orchestrate long-distance strategic 'leaps'. But that is only part of what happens when the rat/flea hypothesis is embraced totally. Benedictow takes the conventional wisdom to its logical conclusion, as follows. If the Black Death really was bubonic plague, he reasons, then, the epidemiology of the disease must be invoked to establish chronologies. The formula used by Benedictow is quite straightforward. First there is the plague among rats. It takes time for an infected rat colony to be decimated and for the fleas to start seeking alternative, human, hosts. Benedictow develops what he calls a 'standard model' for an epidemic to become apparent, viz. it normally takes:

> … 12 days (epizootic) + 3 days (fasting rat fleas) + 0.5-1 (before first infective transmission), 7 days (endemic), + 8 days (incubation and illness for the last endemic cases) + 8 days (incubation and illness for the early epidemic cases infected during the endemic phase), in all 39 days, or 5.6 weeks.[9]

Benedictow even expands this time window by introducing the idea that 'chronicle-producing social élites' would take time to hear about the epidemic that had taken hold in poor communities in bigger towns and cities – possibly seven weeks from the first infestation. The problem is that this all depends on the Black Death *being* bubonic plague. Worse still, it also means that there is never any *record* of the actual date of first arrival of the projected armies of infected rats. It pushes back the whole chronology of the plague and blurs the issue of when plague arrived in particular localities. It makes it difficult to realistically assess rates of spread and to interpret Benedictow's 'metastatic leaps'. All this begs the question: what if the Great Pestilence was not bubonic plague?

HOW TREE-RING RESEARCH HIGHLIGHTS THE FOURTEENTH CENTURY

It could reasonably be asked why a dendrochronologist – someone who studies tree-rings – should be drawn into taking an interest in the fourteenth century. The reason, in this case, was very simple and had nothing to do, in the first instance, with the Black Death. In Ireland, and to an extent in Britain, it proved to be quite difficult to build tree-ring chronologies across the fourteenth century. To put this in context, to build a long tree-ring chronology in a temperate region it is normal to start by studying the ring patterns of living trees and then overlapping those patterns with more ancient patterns derived from buildings or archaeological sites (1). This overlapping procedure is then extended, further and further, back in time. The final result is a continuous year-by-year record of tree growth anchored at the present day by the sampling dates of the living trees.

In the north of Ireland, between 1968 and 1972, the collecting of tree-ring patterns from living oaks, and from building timbers acquired from later medieval houses, castles and archaeological sites, allowed the construction of just such a joined-up chronology from the anchor of the present day back to the 1380s. Samples from living trees gave us the ring patterns back for several centuries, and in Ireland that meant that the longest-lived modern trees had started to grow around 1650. If we had been based in Scotland, or England, we would have been able to find oaks running back to the early or mid-fifteenth century. In that sense we made life difficult for ourselves by trying to build the chronology in Ireland; of course, we only discovered this with hindsight.

Once a living-tree chronology had been established, and checked for internal consistency, the idea was to overlap the growth patterns of wide and narrow rings from the living trees to those from samples from late medieval buildings. As can be imagined, with Irish oaks going back only to around 1650 we had to find oak timbers in buildings from about 1750 in order to provide a sensible overlap of the ring patterns. Unfortunately, the history of Ireland, as regards the exploitation of forests, meant that most of the native oak forests had gone by about 1720.

As a result, it proved impossible to find oak timbers from any mid-eighteenth-century Irish buildings. In fact, the very latest building we ever found, with relevant oak beams, dated only to 1716. This meant that the overlap between the living-tree and the post-medieval chronologies was too short to be statistically robust. This problem resulted in trips to forests, such as Cadzow in Scotland and Sherwood in England. There we built much longer living-tree chronologies – back to 1444 for Cadzow and 1425 for Sherwood. These were then used to check the validity of the short Irish tree-ring overlap. As it turned out, the long Scottish and English chronologies confirmed that we had in fact forged a correct link in our north Irish chronology, even on the basis of the relatively short overlap. The whole exercise, while time consuming, established confidence in our chronology-building procedures. In the long run, this proved very useful in avoiding mistakes further back in time, as the chronology was extended.

So, the reader is now aware that dendrochronologists in Ireland had faced an overlap problem in the late seventeenth century. As we collected more and more oak timbers from seventeenth- and sixteenth-century buildings in the north of Ireland we started to see another problem looming. For example, we found massive oak timbers laid across the River Lagan at Shaw's Bridge, just south of Belfast that had been felled in 1617. When dated, it was found that the centre rings on the oldest samples dated back to 1364 and 1373. As more and more timbers were collected it became clear that all the longest-lived timbers from the seventeenth and sixteenth centuries ran back to the decades following 1350. It began to look as if there was a sort of tree-ring 'wall' in the north of Ireland at about 1350.

As a result, we approached colleagues in the Dublin area and acquired timbers from a series of buildings and late-medieval archaeological contexts around the city. The ring patterns were formed into a Dublin medieval chronology which cross-dated well with the northern chronology. Again, much to our annoyance, the longest-lived timbers had ring patterns that ran *back* only to the 1350s – what, we began to ask, was going on?

The story of how this problem was resolved was published back in the 1970s. At the time we were sampling oaks from many contexts – bogs, river beds, lake edges and archaeological sites – as part of a program aimed at constructing an overall 6000-year tree-ring chronology for radiocarbon calibration purposes. For example, archaeological samples from the Viking and Norman levels in medieval Dublin had provided a chronology which, we now know, spanned AD 855-1306. It did not seem to matter how many more timbers were sampled from the various Dublin excavation sites, that chronology could not be extended any further *forward* in time. In fact, even now, decades later, and with many more timbers dated as part of a commercial dating service, the Dublin chronology still runs up only to 1306. Whatever the reason, be it a change in land use within the city, or truncation of the relevant levels by later cellars, or whatever, something gives rise to a substantial Dublin gap in the fourteenth century from 1306-57. It gradually

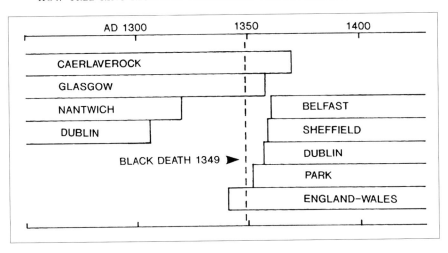

2 The end- and start-dates for various early, British Isles, oak chronologies illustrating the regeneration phase following the Black Death

became clear that there was something peculiar about the survival – rather the non-survival – of oak timbers across the fourteenth century in the wider hinterlands of both Belfast and Dublin. Thus, we were forced to extend our area of sampling and, as luck would have it, timbers were eventually acquired from sites in parts of western Ulster that had been little affected by Norman influence.

In these areas of Irish influence the sites that produced oak timbers were archaeological, particularly crannogs (artificial lake dwellings). These lake platforms often included both oak trunks and worked oak timbers and these formed a useful source of tree-ring samples especially as a number of lakes had their levels lowered in the 1970s, allowing access to sites that were normally submerged. Other assemblages included natural oak trunks dredged from the beds of rivers flowing into Lough Neagh, the large water body in the middle of Northern Ireland. When these assemblages were analysed, and the ring patterns cross-dated, it was found that some provided the essential link across the fourteenth century. To put this work in perspective, it took some seven years of sampling to finally build a chronology back far enough to link with the 1306 Dublin medieval chronology. These linkages gave us a continuous year-by-year record for Irish oak from the present back to 855.

This experience, of trying to build a continuous tree-ring chronology, indicated that the land, or forest, management regime in the west of Ulster was different from that pertaining to the east of Ireland generally. It had to be assumed that the oaks in the east were part of a more highly managed system (with many trees regenerating after 1350) while those from the west conformed better to a model of unmanaged woodland. Having eventually solved the problem of the fourteenth-century 'gap' we could continue on back in time attempting to build the very long,

6000-year, target chronology. However, even though we had successfully 'bridged the fourteenth-century gap' there was an indelible mark, not least in the minds of the dendrochronologists who had been forced to deal with the problem. It was clear that there were *fewer* timbers whose ring patterns spanned the fourteenth century in Ireland compared with the relatively large numbers available from periods before and after. Whether this was due to less timbers being used in the fourteenth century or simply due to their survival rate being different was not altogether clear. However, we can now look back with the benefit of several decades of additional sampling, and review the situation from today's perspective. Here, circumstances allow us to have confidence in the sampling strategy.

Because there is only enough commercial tree-ring dating business to support one dendrochronological laboratory in Ireland, for over 30 years all the oak timbers dug up by archaeologists, or sampled by building historians, have been dated in the Belfast Laboratory. Moreover, because archaeologists, and indeed building historians, seldom know the dates of the samples they excavate or acquire, the Belfast Lab has had the opportunity to date an almost perfectly 'random sample' of the oaks that exist in the ground, or in buildings, throughout the island of Ireland. This has the advantage of providing an almost total picture of the numbers of timbers that exist through time. So, what does this random sampling of oak timbers tell us?

Figure 3 shows the level of replication in the Irish tree-ring record for the fourteenth century. Even after decades of random sampling, it is apparent that there is still a dramatic depletion of timbers in the mid-century. As was originally noted, timbers start growing in large numbers in the later fourteenth century. Even early in the research this was referred to as a 'regeneration' episode. In contrast, the paucity of samples from the decades before 1350, where there were real difficulties in acquiring samples, was referred to as a 'depletion'. The figure indicates this quite well.

It was inevitable that quite early on in this developing story we recognized the close relationship of this widespread tree-ring 'problem' to the plague known as the Black Death that spread to Ireland by 1348 or 1349. If, as was widely stated, this plague killed off about one third of the human population, this offered a possible reason for the observations in the Irish tree-ring work. The first suggested explanation was that the reduction in human population had removed pressure on land and allowed some marginal land to return to forest. In retrospect it is just as likely that there were less people left to manage woodland and the oak regeneration, evident from around 1350, could have been due to reduced management pressure on existing woodlands. The fact that timbers from the west of Ulster seemed not to respect the otherwise widespread depletion/regeneration episode would imply that there was less management of woodlands in the west, something which might fit quite well with the differences between Irish and Norman culture. However, before leaving this replication issue, perhaps we should take a

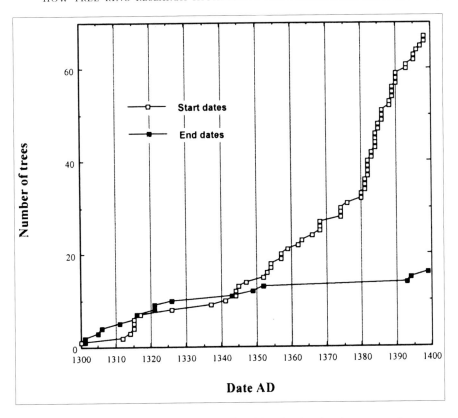

3 All fourteenth-century start- and end-dates for Irish oaks, showing the regeneration excess after 1350. These are running-sum plots used to provide a visual impression of accumulating data. Note the small number of oaks ending and the large number starting in the century

closer look at the plot. It is very clear that the number of timbers felled in the fourteenth century drops almost to nothing by 1350. At the same time we see a change in slope of the plot of start years of the later timbers whose ring patterns run back into the fourteenth century. There are a few trees with start years between 1310 and 1350, but the number increases at a different rate immediately after 1350. What was not originally recognised was the second change of slope that takes place very clearly at 1380. This implies that the story may have some additional complication. It could be that the 1380 increase is merely the post-1350 trees maturing and starting to produce acorns. However, if that were the case it has certain implications for the landscape in which these trees were growing. It might well imply very little human pressure on the regenerating woodlands.

There is a certain power to this sort of observation. We did not set out to study the regeneration pattern of fourteenth-century Irish oaks (we set out only to build a chronology) but we now have a very good picture of that regeneration. The data is inherently powerful because it was randomly sampled; the pattern we now see is unlikely to change even with further sampling. So it is probably a real reflection of one aspect of what was going on in Ireland in the later fourteenth century – it seems that there was nothing in the landscape to inhibit oak regeneration.

As mentioned previously, in the 1970s we undertook the construction of a long oak chronology in Scotland in order to independently replicate the whole of the last 1000 years of the Irish chronology. In part this was an insurance exercise because we were concerned that the fourteenth-century section of the Irish chronology might be inherently weak, and it might not prove possible to bridge the fourteenth-century gap. As it happened, Scotland presented a completely different picture from the one observed in Ireland. Overall, in Scotland, chronology building ran like clockwork. Whereas in Ireland it had taken from 1968-77 to produce 1000 years of chronology, in Scotland the same length of chronology was achieved in a matter of months. To paraphrase the procedure:

Lockwood modern oak ring patterns ran back to 1571
Cadzow modern oak ring patterns ran back to 1444
Castle of Park timbers gave ring patterns spanning 1551-1350
Lincluden oak panels gave ring patterns spanning 1467-1068
Glasgow Cathedral oak beams gave ring patterns spanning 1360-946[1]

What was immediately apparent was the appearance of the dates 1350 and 1360, associated with the *inner rings* from Castle of Park and the *outer rings* from Glasgow Cathedral. Obviously, if the Lincluden panels had not been acquired, we would have had a 'gap' (in tree-ring terms a 10-year overlap is the same as a gap because no linkage could be established on such a short overlap) at 1350 in Scotland as well as in Ireland. This straightforward chronology building exercise indicated that the same fourteenth-century depletion/regeneration episode we had deduced in Ireland was also evident in Scotland.

It is possible to elaborate further on the issue of the later fourteenth-century regeneration. Part of the stimulus for the work in Scotland had been a request from archaeologist Chris Tabraham that we investigate the dating of the timber bridges from the moat of the famous triangular castle at Caerlaverock, near Dumfries. A series of oak foundations for timber bridges had been found in the moat during excavations in the 1960s. These timbers had been replaced in 'the hope of future dendrochronology'.[2] So, a mere decade after the original excavations – while we were constructing the Scottish chronology – the moat was drained and the timbers sampled for dating. The results were interesting in several ways, but one in particular is relevant here. There were four phases of timbering in the moat and three of these provided long-lived oaks that dated easily against the Scottish chronology indicating felling phases (i) around 1277, (ii) in 1333, and (iii) in 1371. So here was another case of long-lived oaks running into the fourteenth century but failing to bridge right across the century.

This left the fourth phase of timbering. These timbers were completely different in terms of their growth character. Although they were large in cross section, they had only a few very wide growth rings; the maximum number of rings in any of the timbers was only 59, which is less than any acceptable minimum for dating purposes (in our experience). They were not datable by using dendrochronology. (For those not familiar with dendrochronology the ring pattern of a sample is compared with a relevant master chronology at every possible position of overlap, looking for a position with significant agreement. A short pattern – anything with significantly less than 100 rings – usually cannot be uniquely dated because its pattern will tend to match at a number of different positions.) However, a combination of detailed radiocarbon analysis and relevant building history showed that the timbers had been growing in the early fifteenth century and had been felled close to 1450.[3] So at Caerlaverock Castle we were seeing a change in character in the timbers after the mid-fourteenth century. Whereas all the timbers felled in the phases up to 1370 had been long lived (each typically more than 200 years old), those felled in the early to mid-fifteenth century were wide ringed and fast grown – rapidly-regenerating young trees. Examples like this serve to reinforce the whole regeneration picture. When we find oak building timbers felled in the early fifteenth century they are not from the same population of long-lived timbers used up to 1350, they are from a new, regenerated stock.

Overall, building oak chronologies in Ireland and Scotland had demonstrated that in eastern Ireland and in Scotland there was essentially a 'gap' centred on 1350. That gap seemed to be marked by the end of long-lived timbers followed by the rapid regeneration of young trees. We were able to find hints of the same thing in England where two chronologies had been constructed that started in the mid-fourteenth century; one spanned 1341-1636,[4] the other 1359-1591.[5] Thus the regeneration that occurred in the mid-fourteenth-century could be claimed to be widespread in the British Isles.

The upshot of these various observations was that there seemed to be, within the British Isles, a definite tree response to the Black Death. We could have left the issue there but because other workers were also dating a lot of buildings in other countries, it was not long before we noted a building hiatus in Germany beginning in 1347. In 1980 Ernst Hollstein produced a detailed study of the results of his career in dating oak timbers from buildings in Germany.[6] The results were fascinating. In one diagram Hollstein drew up a record of all the buildings and archaeological sites he had dated.

The easiest way to describe this is as follows. Hollstein found no timbers that dated between 966 and 1038; so it was clear that you could have periods where not enough building was going on to provide samples to the present day. Following this 71-year gap, from 1038-1347 Hollstein found, on average, one datable timber or structure every nine years (33 sites, phases, or structures, in 310 years). Then quite abruptly, at 1347, the dates stop and no further dated structures are found until after 1425.

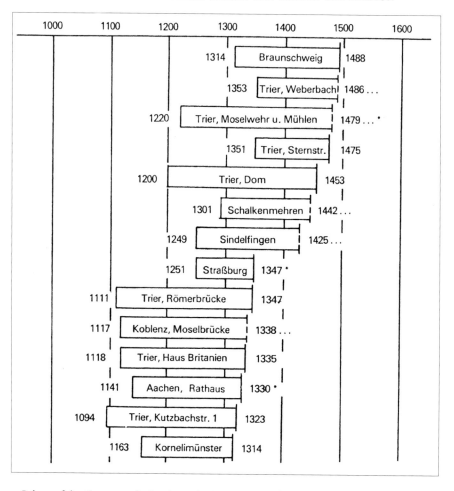

4 Subset of the German oak site chronologies constructed by Ernst Hollstein showing the building hiatus from 1347 to c.1440[7]

Just at the time when the Black Death arrives into Europe, we see a change from a date every nine years to an interval of some 80 years with no building. Then from 1425–1679 the rate returns to one date every eight years. Given that, as noted previously, the dating of sites/buildings is a quasi-random procedure – simply because in most cases the date is unknown before the analysis is undertaken – this suite of results highlights the direct impact of the Black Death in Germany immediately after 1347. In fact the picture has been replicated almost exactly in work carried out by Burghart Schmidt dating houses in the Mosel area.[8] Again, as soon as Peter Kuniholm started dating buildings in Greece he found a broadly similar result with buildings up to 1347 and fewer buildings thereafter.[9]

With these tree-ring findings from the British Isles, through Germany, to Greece, the implication is that, even if we had no written history, dendrochronologists would have been forced to ask what vector could cause a depletion/regeneration in the British Isles and a building hiatus from Germany to Greece, all at the same time? It would not have taken a genius to suggest that a possible explanation would be a pandemic i.e. it seems possible that dendrochronologists could have detected the effects of the Black Death even if no human records had been in existence. This of course hints at the power of dendrochronology to uncover events through the simple act of dating lots of structures. It alerts us to look at any breaks in regular sequences of building in the more distant past as possible clues to reductions in human population.

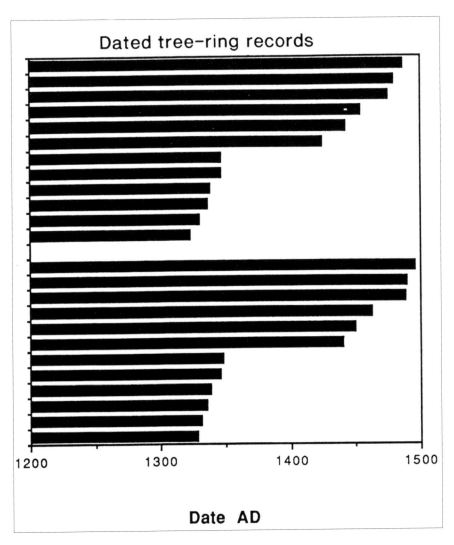

5 Building hiatus following 1347 in both the Aegean (Peter Kuniholm)[9] and Germany (Ernst Hollstein)[6]

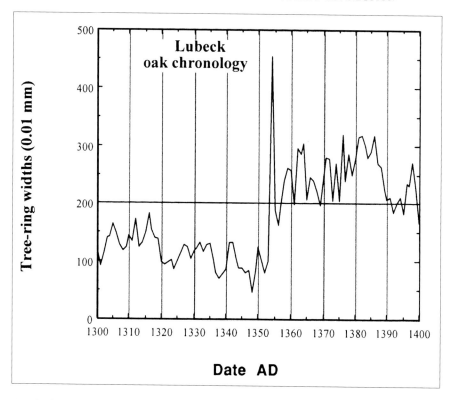

6 Oak chronology from Lubeck, Germany, showing the ring-width 'step' after 1350 due to the change from old narrow-ringed trees to young regenerating trees. *Data courtesy Sigrid Wrobel*

Before leaving this initial tree-ring introduction it is worth pointing out just how extreme this sort of effect can be. At Lubeck, in north Germany, dendrochronologists from Hamburg were constructing a chronology. What they found there was the use of long-lived, narrow-ringed, oaks up to 1350. Thereafter, the next section of chronology comprised oaks felled in later centuries that had started growing just at 1350. When a mean chronology is plotted there is a huge 'step' in ring width as one goes from the narrow-ringed old material to the wide-ringed young trees after 1350. This step is, of course, an indelible reminder of the arrival of the plague in north Germany.

CONCLUSION

From quite early in the story of European dendrochronology it was apparent that the fourteenth century was interesting and that the Black Death had had real tangible effects on timber survival. It is important to stress again that the fourteenth century was only a problem in the initial chronology building process. Once the gap was bridged that problem had gone; however, the legacy is still a clear depletion in the number of samples.

The two changes in slope in the regenerating Irish oaks at 1350 and 1380 were highlighted in *Figure 3*. Looked at again it is clear that *most* of the sixteenth- and seventeenth-century timbers sampled by dendrochronologists had started growing not after 1350 but after 1380. This raises a number of questions. Possible solutions that might be worth considering would be a secondary environmental event of some kind around 1380. The possibility has already been mentioned of the oaks regenerating after 1350 producing acorns for the first time in the 1380s. However is it possible that the observation of more trees regenerating after 1380 is giving a hint that something caused a reduction in grazing pressure by pigs, or other animals, due to something affecting the animal populations; a murrain perhaps? As usual with the past there is little to go on in trying to provide a definitive answer. The observation at this stage is simply 'interesting'. However, it might be worth keeping an eye out for anything strange in the 1380s.

2

THE GLOBAL PICTURE

Dendrochronologists do not normally think in terms of widespread regional sig-nal; still less in terms of a 'global' signal. By definition, tree-ring workers have to construct their chronologies on a relatively local basis. In fact, there is strong pressure on any dendrochronologist setting out to build a chronology to think on as small a geographical scale as possible. This is because it limits the number of variables that have to be taken into account. For example, in Ireland, the initial chronological work was carried out in the north of the island within about a 50-mile radius of Lough Neagh. This meant that all the oaks collected tended to have grown in a similar climate regime somewhat sheltered from the prevailing winds from the Atlantic. Only later, as it became obvious that we could cross-date ring patterns from the north of Ireland to those from the Dublin region, and Scotland, did we start to broaden our horizons and accept that we could use trees from a wider area in our chronologies.

As a result of this local approach, it was inevitable that, in Europe, we ended up with many locally based – Irish, Scottish, north English, south English, north German, south German, Polish etc. – chronologies. We have seen already (Chapter 1) how the internal integrity of the Irish chronology, for the last 1000 years, was tested by constructing a Scottish chronology. Grids of chronologies also allow third-level replication, where chronologies constructed by different workers, in different laboratories, in different areas, can be checked one against the other. It was during such inter-regional comparisons that it started to become clear that a strong matching component (governing oak growth) existed right across northern Europe from Ireland to Poland. That is, although each of the chro-nologies was built separately (on the initial assumption that there would be little agreement between regions) in fact quite strong agreement existed between oak chronologies even from distant locations.

Once these numerous regional chronologies were available, use could be made of them for comparison and replication purposes. In fact, having a widespread grid of local chronologies allows dendrochronologists to provenance samples of imported or traded wood. With a grid of chronologies available, a new sample can be compared with all the chronologies. Often it is possible to contour the resulting correlation values so that the original location where the sample grew can be defined quite closely. One excellent example is Skuldelev II, one of the Viking-period, Roskilde block-ships, found in a fjord in Denmark. When the ring patterns of its timbers were compared with all the medieval chronologies from northern Europe it was found that the highest correlations contoured onto Ireland. This indicated that the ship was constructed in Ireland, around AD 1060, using oak timbers from a region close to the city of Dublin.[1]

While that level of progression from local to regional to pan-European sounds perfectly logical, historically it is important to realize that some early observations had served to cloud the issue of regional cross-matching signal. In the 1970s a suite of what were called 'art-historical' chronologies were constructed in England and

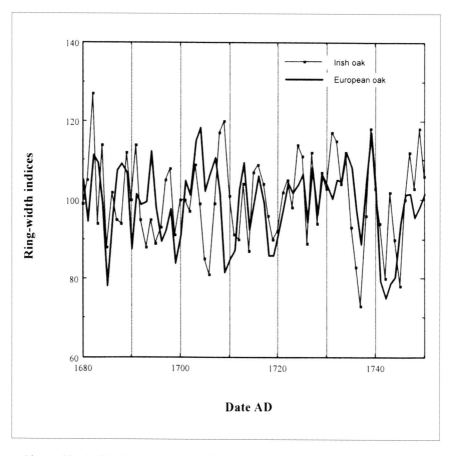

7 Observed level of similarity between the Irish oak chronology and an average European oak chronology

the Netherlands. These used mostly oak panels that had served as the supports for late medieval oil paintings. It was observed that the art-historical chronologies constructed in England cross-dated with similar art-historical chronologies built in the Netherlands; however, they both singularly failed to cross match with any of the main regional chronologies from Germany or the British Isles that were available during the 1970s. The English art-historical chronologies in particular were claimed, with strongly presented arguments, to be composed of oaks that had grown in England but which were somehow 'different'.[2] These observations served to cloud the issue of common signal between oak chronologies – apparently there were geographic pockets where the chronologies were obeying some different signal. It was only after a good deal of skirmishing around the various issues involved in the debate that it was proven that these particular 'English' oaks had grown in the eastern Baltic region and had come into England as part of Hansa, and later, trade. An exactly similar situation was indicated for many of the oak boards used for paintings in the Low Countries. Only when this issue was satisfactorily resolved, in the mid-1980s, did it become fully apparent just how much common tree-ring signal existed across northern Europe.[3]

An easy way to demonstrate the existence of this common signal in oak tree-rings is by making up two independent chronologies. Quite arbitrarily we looked at 14 available oak chronologies from northern Europe. We left out the Lubeck chronology for the reasons given in association with *Figure 6*; that left 13 chronologies. We picked seven from north, west and south Germany, the Netherlands, southern and eastern England, and Ireland and averaged them together. We then did the same thing for the remaining six chronologies from Poland, Denmark, north Germany, southern and northern England and Scotland. *Figure 8* shows the resulting pattern. It is very clear that the two average chronologies are very similar. In a sense it did not matter which chronologies were used or indeed where the chronologies were built. As soon as any six or seven chronologies are available their average is a stable representation of the *common signal*. Build any other half dozen oak chronologies anywhere from Ireland to Poland and essentially the same average chronology will appear. Most people are not aware of just how robust a system dendrochronology is, but this averaging approach shows what a consistent a story the oaks are recording.

Now there is some irony in this observation. Because dendrochronology works *so* well, it is clear that the oaks across Europe are recording this 'common signal'. It would be reasonable, if a strong signal is being recorded, to assume that we should be able to extract it from the chronologies. The irony is that in attempts to extract climate signal from oak chronologies only some 25-40 per cent of the variation in the ring widths can be accounted for by temperature and rainfall records. We are left with the fact that the oaks know pretty much what to do each year in terms of growth; however, there are more factors influencing that growth than just temperature and rainfall.

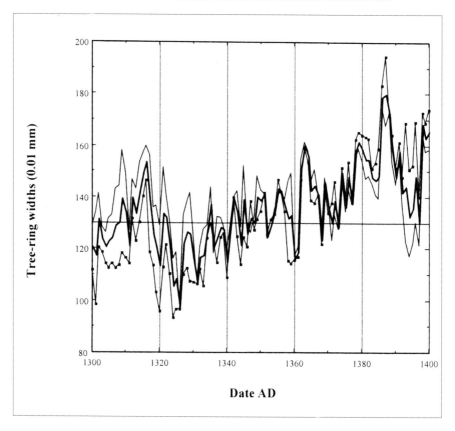

8 Two totally independent, average, European oak chronologies plotted with the overall average chronology showing very similar year-to-year detail. The growth depression in the 1320s and 1330s is clearly evident

Overall, we can say that tree-ring patterns match well because of response to a common climatic signal, yet it is difficult to extract that signal from the ring patterns.

From the point of view of this book, attempting to make some sense of the environment of the fourteenth century, it is interesting to take a look at the overall European oak chronology. *Figure 9* shows the 13-site chronology from *Figure 8* plotted at annual resolution and with a 5-point smoothed version superimposed to highlight the trends in the data.

Looking at *Figure 9* it is very evident that there were significant reductions in European oak growth in the 1320s and 1330s. It would be nice to have some hint of what may have caused these responses by the oak trees. Looking around for relevant information it was observed that other workers had noted a sudden cooling of the North Atlantic surface water, simultaneous with the abrupt downturn in European oak growth. This information was provided by

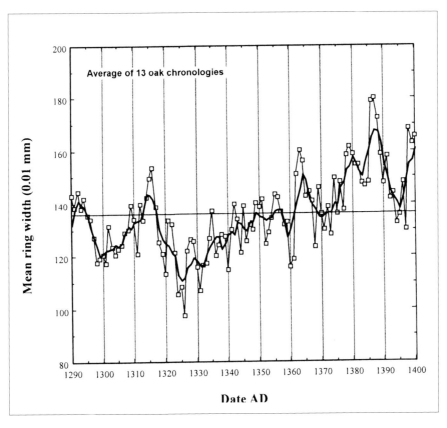

9 The average of 13 oak chronologies from Ireland to Poland showing oak growth across northern Europe AD 1290-1400

the environmentalist Alistair Dawson, who was working on the issue of North Atlantic sea-surface temperatures (NAsst). These temperatures are derived from measurements on the stable isotopes of oxygen in the Greenland ice. The method is elegant and requires a little explanation. The heavy isotope of hydrogen is deuterium. During cold conditions it is slightly harder to lift water made with the heavy isotope from the ocean surface. So, when it is cold the water vapour from the oceans, falling as snow in Greenland, is *depleted* in deuterium. By analysing the deuterium record, preserved in the layers of compressed snowfall in the ice cores, it is possible to reconstruct a temperature record, at annual resolution, far back in time.

When we plot this sea-surface temperature reconstruction with European oak-ring widths (*10*) it is apparent that the reduction in European oak growth tracks the reductions in NAsst very closely. This implies very strongly that for this period, at least, the oaks were responding to changes in temperature in the North Atlantic region. One particularly good thing about working in the fourteenth

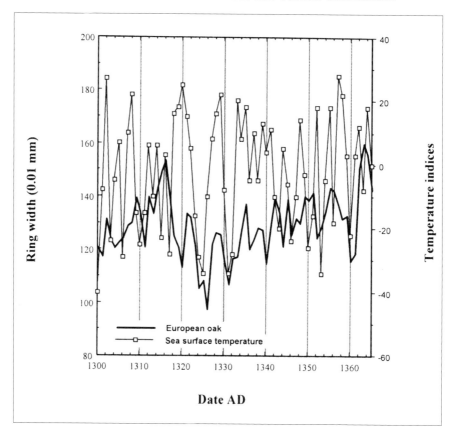

10 North Atlantic estimated sea surface temperature plotted with the 13-site European average oak chronology from *Figure 8*. Showing a possible link in reduced growth with reduced temperature in the 1320s and 1330s. *Sea surface temperature data courtesy Alistair Dawson*

century is that we have a check on the accuracy of the ice-core dating. We know that it is possible to locate, and identify, tephra (volcanic glass) shards from a specific Icelandic volcanic eruption, Öraefajokull, that took place in 1362. For example, in the GRIP ice core, the glass shards occur specifically in the ice layer dated to 1362 by detailed layer counting.[4] With this information we now know that we can make direct tree-ice comparisons.

We now have a coherent set of oak tree-ring chronologies for northern Europe. Imagine that, as a dendrochronologist, you were accumulating these regional chronologies and comparing them. You may be looking for periods when they either all react similarly or, as they sometimes do, act differently. Doing this in the 1990s, it quickly became apparent that there were some common regional elements in the chronologies. For example, it was obvious that there were significant growth downturns in the 1740s and the 1320s in European oak; it seemed sensible to cast around to see what was happening in other chronologies. Here we run

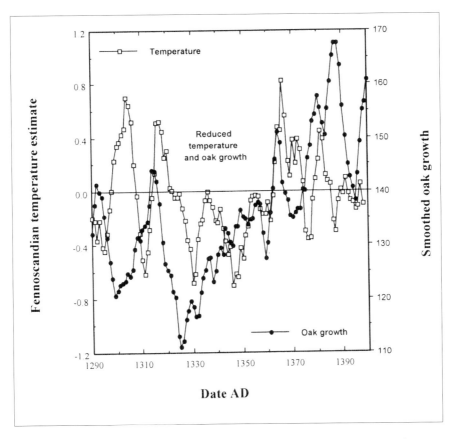

11 Comparison of a 5-point smoothed version of the European oak chronology with a temperature reconstruction from Fennoscandian pine[5] again indicating reduced oak growth coincident with reduced temperature 1320-50

into the benefit of a small discipline like dendrochronology, where data exchange is common between protagonists. Workers in Fennoscandia, particularly Hakan Grudd, had been constructing pine chronologies in northern areas where the trees are sensitive to summer temperature. Such chronologies excite dendro-climatologists, such as Keith Briffa at the Climatic Research Unit at Norwich, because they allow the possibility of reconstructing past summer temperatures.[6] These workers had kindly made their temperature record, deduced from the densities and widths of Swedish pines, available; so they can be plotted against the oak record for comparison. *Figure 11* shows the plot of the two records across the fourteenth century. It is immediately apparent that there is a growth downturn, in this case *at least partially temperature related*, in both records. Two different species of tree in different geographical regions both recorded something happening in the run-up to the Black Death. Examination of the tree-ring graphs in *Figure 11* shows that both chronologies were still indicating below average growth through

to 1350. This was the first indication that the Black Death had a definite environmental context. The late 1340s were not just an arbitrary point in time, when a
plague 'just happened' to arrive. To put it simply, the Black Death sits in an environmental trough when European trees were registering below-normal growth.

That figure was published in 1996. Shortly thereafter, on a research visit to New
Zealand, Chung Limin entered the picture. Chung had just completed a PhD on
the dendroclimatology of New Zealand cedar. In the course of this work he had
updated old chronologies built in the 1970s by Val LaMarche from Tucson, and
built a suite of new cedar chronologies. In the end he had 23 chronologies from
a range of sites and altitudes across New Zealand. With the European experience
as background, Chung was introduced to the idea of adding the chronologies
together to look for common signal. When this was done the surprising finding

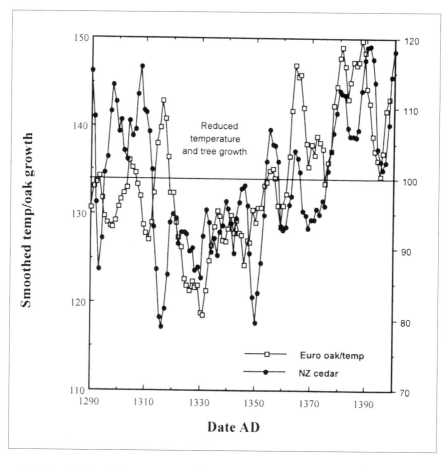

12 Combined oak and pine temperature from *Figure 11* plotted with an average New
Zealand cedar chronology (both smoothed) showing the coincident reduced growth/
temperature 1320-50

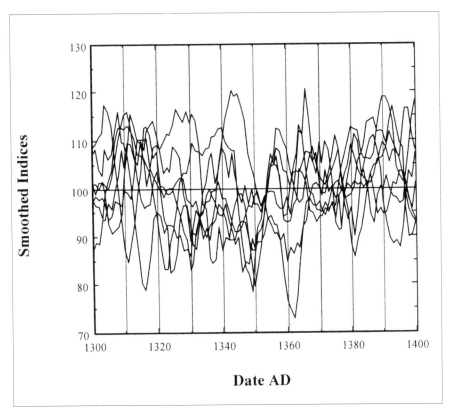

13 Eight smoothed tree-ring chronologies from around the world showing expected noisy behaviour, with a suggestion of a downturn around 1350

was that the master cedar chronology showed a series of growth downturns that were familiar from the European oak work. Remember that dendrochronologists tend to think locally, there are no grounds for expecting to see similar patterns on exactly opposite sides of the planet! Yet it was apparent that the New Zealand tree-ring patterns presented the same well-known growth downturns at AD 1740, at AD 1601, and in the fourteenth century, that had already been seen in the Irish/ European work, see *Figure 12*. When trees on opposite sides of the world pick up similar patterns then they must be responding to some elements of *global* signal. This was the first hint that the happenings in the fourteenth century might not just be European; they might be part of some global pattern.

This observation led to a search for some more widespread chronologies. Almost immediately it was possible to acquire some eight regional chronologies from around the world. The first was the European oak chronology; this chronology was the average of a series of oak chronologies, from a region spanning Ireland to Poland. Notice that in this case the entire European oak record is reduced to a single common curve, presumably representing the mean growth response of tens of millions of oaks. Then there was the Fennoscandian chronology from Hakan Grudd. Keith Briffa kindly provided a chronology from the Polar Urals constructed by Stepan Shiyatov and Eugene Vaganov. Don Graybill originally sent the data for nine bristlecone pine chronologies (also available from the Tucson Laboratory for Tree-Ring Research at Tucson). Again these were meaned into one representative bristlecone chronology for the western United States. Peter Kuniholm provided three replicated chronologies from the Aegean. Antonio Lara provided chronologies from South America and Ed Cook provided a huon pine chronology from Tasmania. That is a pretty big assemblage of tree-ring data and it is probably fair to say that as a first approximation it is representative of temperate tree-growth worldwide. So what does it look like?

Figure 13 shows the eight chronologies plotted on the same time axis. As might be expected with tree populations from differing climate regimes around the world the picture is pretty chaotic. However, one way to clarify things is by lumping data together to form broad regional groupings. These are then plotted as averages of four Old World chronologies and four non-Old World

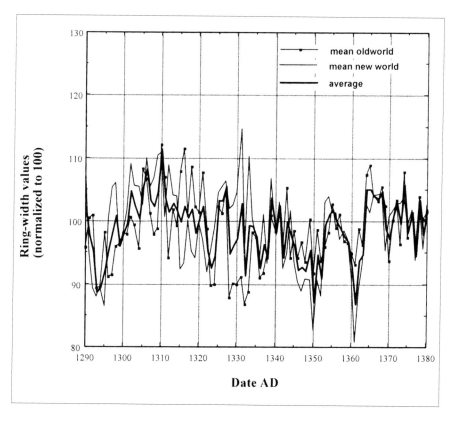

14 Annual resolution chronologies (four from the Old World and four non-Old World) and the overall average (heavy line) 1290–1400

chronologies as in *Figure 14*. Then, to see the general trend of what is going on through the fog of annual resolution data the chronologies can be smoothed as illustrated in *Figure 15*.

It is important for the reader to realize a basic fact about all this. When these graphs were plotted it was the first time anyone had ever had the opportunity to view a 'global' tree-ring chronology. To be able to do so placed dendrochronologists in Belfast in a strangely privileged position. It was as if, for the first time, there was a well-dated 'history' according to the trees. Looking at these figures, it is immediately apparent that all the curves are below 100 per cent in the 1340s and again in the early 1360s. This confirmed what was hinted at originally in the European oak and pine chronologies. The Black Death sits in a clear environmental trough visible in smoothed tree-ring chronologies from around the world.

In *Figures 14* and *15* we see that at the start of the century the two chronologies are doing similar things. Then between 1310 and 1335 we see dramatically opposite activity between the two hemispheric chronologies. Perhaps most surprising is that after 1335 we see both chronologies again behaving in parallel. Then, not

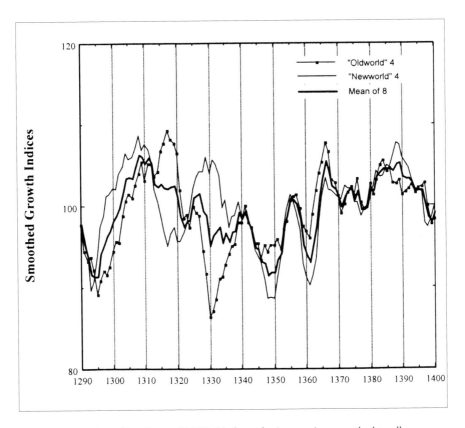

15 The same Old World and non-Old World chronologies 5-point smoothed to allow comparison of the trends in the data

only are the chronologies similar in the second half of the fourteenth century, they are *ridiculously* similar. No one would have expected trees in opposite hemispheres to show such similar growth responses. Clearly, after 1350, something is forcing the world's temperate trees to behave in a remarkably similar way. There are a limited number of factors that can force such a global response.

CONCLUSION

What can we conclude from this chapter? We can immediately recognize that the Black Death has a clear environmental context. The Black Death sits in a global tree-ring trough which must have been caused by some robust forcing agent changing to produce widespread reduced growth in trees – a piece of information previously missing from the historical record. One could be forgiven for wondering if crops may have suffered in the same way. For example, if the forcing agent was the sun, then reduced sunlight could have resulted in a global growth reduction including food crops as well as a global reduction in tree growth. But it is also inescapable that there was a reduction in the human population of a good part of the Old World in the 1340s (and quite possibly beyond). Are we seeing something like – less tree growth … less crop yields … less humans – a sort of global productivity reduction?

The other surprising finding is the remarkably similar growth response between the hemispheres in the second half of the fourteenth century. In particular, all the chronologies climb out of the later 1340s together. Now obviously this is a bit of an oversimplification, because we do not have all the chronologies in the world, we just have eight. However, it would be reasonable, if one were giving a talk on this issue, to simplify the statement down to something like 'How would you get 'all the trees in the world' to do the same thing at the same time'? Yes, indeed, how would you? You would have to start thinking about issues such as giving them more sunlight or rainfall (but rainfall should not work because of the quite strong regional differences in rainfall patterns around the world). Alternatively you might give them more CO_2 so that they grow better (that might work). But, it is possible to play mind games with this. Imagine that you somehow release some extra CO_2 to allow trees to grow better; where could that CO_2 come from? One obvious source is the methane stored as clathrate in the sea-beds off continental margins. It is estimated that there may be 10,000 gigatons of carbon stored as CH_4 (methane) in this way. If some of this were to be released and converted by burning to CO_2, that might produce a short greenhouse pulse, enough to stimulate tree-growth. In fact it probably would not be necessary to burn the methane. Methane is itself a greenhouse gas, maybe all that is necessary to explain the observations would be a large methane release. Or, again, the easiest way to get all trees to grow better is to fertilize them in some way. Is there a mechanism for dumping a fertilizer like ammonia into the earth's atmosphere? It turns out that there are several possible mechanisms! If a number of bolides explode in the atmosphere, these should produce ammonia which could easily act as a general fertilizer. Or again, massive forest fires are believed to leave ammonium layers in the Greenland ice record. Could that source of ammonia act to fertilize all the trees? Wait a minute, forest fires could in theory initially screen out the sun by forming a 'dust' (soot) veil, something that could account for the reduced tree growth. Then as the ammonium settles or rains out it could act as a fertilizer. That almost sounds plausible. Where could we look for some evidence that might shed light on that possibility – obviously the ice cores? We shall come back to this later.

What this speculative excursion demonstrates is this: by simply identifying what trees were doing around the world in the mid-fourteenth century, a whole new suite of questions is opened up. We can start asking questions about issues as diverse as clathrates (gas-bearing ices that occur under certain conditions of temperature and pressure, in buried layers on the continental shelves). This question, in itself, raises the issue of earthquakes, because an earthquake would be the most likely cause of a gas release. Such thoughts, in turn, raise the question of impacts from space; because impacts can trigger earthquakes. What about comets? Could impacting comet fragments deposit material *directly* into the earth's atmosphere? Notice that we can start asking these questions even before we have looked for additional evidence. What we are seeing is the tree-ring chronologies acting as a springboard for research ideas. There is no doubt that the questions raised by the tree-ring downturn in the 1340s require answers.

Ammonia: to clarify terminology, when it is in the atmosphere we refer to ammonia gas; when it is deposited in, say, Greenland ice, it is a salt of ammonia, most probably ammonium hydroxide or ammonium nitrate, and it is referred to as ammonium.

3

THE RADIOCARBON STORY

We have now seen that tree-ring chronologies suggest some environmental changes taking place in the fourteenth century. The importance of dendrochronology lies in its absolute dating precision. Tree-ring samples were used to underpin the calibration of the radiocarbon time-scale. This means that it is worth looking to see what was happening to the radioactive carbon trace gas in the atmosphere at the same time. In this chapter we will see that there are interesting hints in the radiocarbon record of changes taking place in the run-up to the Black Death.

Willard Libby developed the radiocarbon dating method back in the late 1940s and was subsequently awarded a Nobel Prize. The leap of logic that led to this important scientific breakthrough in the field of chronology was breathtaking in its own way. Libby hypothesised that ^{14}C, the radioactive isotope of normal ^{12}C, was only formed as a by-product of cosmic ray interaction with ^{14}N in the earth's atmosphere (the cosmic rays are from deep space). He also hypothesised that this cosmogenic radioactive isotope of carbon would then mix with the normal ^{12}C in the atmosphere and would be taken up by everything in the biosphere, whether plant or animal (plants take carbon in from the atmosphere during photosynthesis, animals get their carbon from eating plants or animals that ate plants). So Libby predicted that the whole biosphere (with rare exceptions) would contain a ratio of ^{14}C to ^{12}C which is in balance with the proportion in the atmosphere. Libby also realized that this situation would only apply while the plant or animal was alive. Once anything organic dies, it stops being in balance with the atmosphere and the amount of radiocarbon begins to decrease through radioactive decay. This process is extremely regular and the decay rate of ^{14}C is known. In fact, the time it takes for half of any given number of radioactive ^{14}C atoms to decay back to nitrogen is 5730 years. So Libby obtained his Nobel Prize for realizing that if you measure how much radiocarbon is left in an old organic sample you can work out how much time has elapsed since the organism was alive by the following formula:

Time since death = function (half-life ^{14}C) x function (remaining proportion
^{14}C/^{12}C)

The problem was that, back in the 1940s, Libby had to make an important assumption. For the radiocarbon method to work, he had to assume that the proportion of ^{14}C to ^{12}C in the atmosphere had always been the same i.e. that all living material *always* had the same proportion of ^{14}C to ^{12}C while alive. There was not much he could do about this other than do some rough and ready checks. He obtained samples of known-age organic material from Egypt, and elsewhere, and measured their radiocarbon ages. He found that his scientific dates were 'pretty much in line' with the known ages, and he felt justified in going ahead with applying the dating method to real research questions. That was fine for about 20 years, but gradually it became clear to customers, e.g. archaeologists purchasing dates, that something was not quite right. There was a tendency for known-age samples from Egypt or the Aegean to be consistently a bit too young compared with their known ages. It was at this point, in the later 1960s, that people moved to testing Libby's theory empirically. This could be done by taking consecutive samples of wood from long American tree-ring chronologies. These samples were exactly dated by dendrochronology. By measuring their radiocarbon age it would be possible to see any deviation from the true age. This process in science is known as calibration – the checking of a method against a known standard. In this case the tree-ring samples represent the precisely dated standard, against which the radiocarbon method is being checked.

This work was first carried out in America and the resultant calibration curve was produced by Hans Suess.[1] It showed that Libby's theory was pretty good but not perfect. As one goes back in time, beyond about 500 BC, radiocarbon dates become systematically too young compared with real dates. By 6000 years ago the discrepancy is almost 1000 years. None of this was fatal for Libby's theory because one could use Suess's calibration curve to correct the raw Libby dates – an excellent application of science.

There were a couple of snags however. First, it was noticed during the calibration exercise that there were short-term fluctuations in the calibration curve. This led to some difficulties in interpreting dates and to arguments as to whether the fluctuations were real – some critics suggested that the fluctuations (Suess had called them 'wiggles') were just statistical noise associated with the measurement process. Second, it was argued that the Suess curve was American and mostly based on trees (bristlecone pines) that had grown at high altitudes. Some workers said that you could not, or should not, use a high-altitude American calibration curve to correct low-altitude Old World radiocarbon dates, i.e. in their view the curve was only valid in America. Because of these various quibbles it was inevitable that the whole calibration exercise would have to be done again, this time using low-altitude Old World samples. Hence the construction of the Irish oak chronology, and to some extent the construction of the central German oak chronology, both of which were used extensively for radiocarbon calibration purposes.

This means that the scientific community have a large number of high-quality radiocarbon measurements on samples of precisely dated wood from all periods back for several thousands of years. Thus, if we want to look for changes in the amount of radiocarbon in the atmosphere through time, indeed at any particular period of time, we can consult the radiocarbon calibration curves. An obvious question is 'what do the radiocarbon calibration curves show in the fourteenth century?' It turns out that what they show is every bit as interesting as the tree-ring evidence.

The construction of an oak chronology in Ireland was specifically aimed at the calibration of the radiocarbon timescale. Not only was a 7000-year oak chronology constructed, but it was checked against oak chronologies from Germany. At the same time, during the 1970s, major efforts were made to improve the precision of the radiocarbon measurements. By the mid-1980s Gordon Pearson, at Belfast, and Minze Stuiver, at Seattle, had both produced calibration datasets.[2]

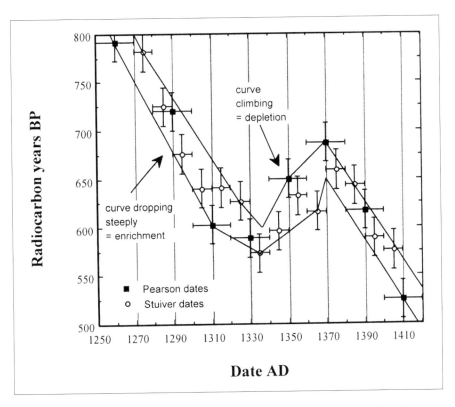

16 The radiocarbon calibration measurements by Gordon Pearson (on Irish oak) and Minze Stuiver (on American pine) across the fourteenth century showing the change from enrichment to depletion in the atmosphere

The results were so similar that the two curves were combined into a single internationally agreed calibration curve. Where did this leave the Suess controversy? It turned out that Suess had been broadly correct all along. There were short-term fluctuations or 'wiggles' in the new replicated calibrations and the overall shape of the curve was similar in both the Old and New Worlds. So, why not retain the Suess curve? In reality the new high-precision datasets were quite simply *better* than the results produced by Suess – a whole new generation of radiocarbon technology had rendered the Suess results obsolete (a good analogue would be the difference between valves and transistors).

With the calibration curves available, we can look with some confidence at how the reservoir of radiocarbon in the atmosphere was changing through time. When we look at the Stuiver/Pearson calibration datasets across the fourteenth century (16) we see that there had been a long period of radiocarbon enrichment from the middle of the thirteenth century – enrichment indicating that more radiocarbon was being produced than Libby's theory would have suggested. More radiocarbon production means that radiocarbon dates are getting *younger*, faster. That long period of enrichment suggests that something is affecting the flux of cosmic radiation arriving at the earth's atmosphere. The conventional wisdom is that the cosmic ray flux from deep space is more or less constant, so something must have been affecting the cosmic radiation at that time. That something is believed to be the sun – to be precise, the solar wind. When the sun is active, the solar wind tends to push away a component of the cosmic radiation arriving into the inner solar system. With less cosmic radiation striking the earth's atmosphere, less radiocarbon will be produced; conversely, when the sun is quiet there is less solar wind so more cosmic radiation arrives producing more radiocarbon.

So, just by looking at the radiocarbon calibration results we can infer that from the mid-thirteenth century, down to about 1335, there was continuous radiocarbon enrichment and therefore the sun should have been relatively quiet. Then, fairly abruptly after 1330 the enrichment ceases and the calibration curve changes direction, the atmospheric reservoir going from enrichment (where more ^{14}C is being produced) to depletion (where the reservoir is being diluted by old carbon, i.e. carbon containing less ^{14}C). Depletion is interesting because to deplete the amount of radiocarbon in the atmosphere it is not sufficient merely to turn down, or even switch off, radiocarbon production. In order for the calibration curve to deplete steeply, i.e. for radiocarbon dates to get rapidly older (as we see some time after 1335) something has to be *diluting* the amount of radiocarbon in the atmosphere. That something has to be 'old' carbon, i.e. carbon with a higher proportion of ^{12}C to ^{14}C. There are several possible sources for old carbon, from comets to volcanoes to ocean-bed clathrates (as noted, clathrates are ice matrices that hold gas under certain conditions of temperature and pressure in the sea bed), but the most likely is probably some sort of overturn of the oceans bringing old water with depleted levels of ^{14}C up to the ocean surface and hence into the atmosphere.

Going back to the calibration, the Stuiver/Pearson data is pretty good but it turns out that there is an even more refined calibration dataset available. For some years radiocarbon laboratories in Waikato, New Zealand, and Belfast, Ireland, have been simultaneously measuring the radiocarbon ages of samples of wood of exactly the same calendar age from both British Isles oak and from New Zealand cedar.[3] *Figure 17* shows the replicated results. To put this in perspective, this is the most thorough calibration exercise ever carried out. Part of the reason for undertaking this exhaustive work was to look at changes in the hemispheric radiocarbon offset through time (it has always been known that there is an offset between the hemispheres; this work was to trace it systematically through time). In the replicated figure we see exactly the same change from enrichment to depletion of radiocarbon as was apparent in the original Stuiver/Pearson results. However, we can have much more confidence in this replicated dataset.

Notice, depending on whose data one uses, a very slightly different picture emerges.

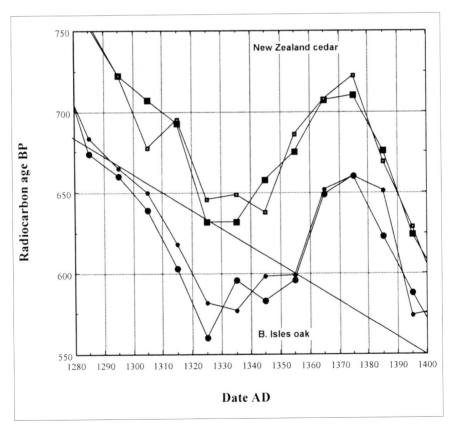

17 Fully replicated, parallel, calibration curves by Gerry McCormac on British Isles oak and Alan Hogg on New Zealand cedar showing a more refined version of *Figure 16*

Suess – was simply not refined enough across the fourteenth century to be any use

Stuiver (10-ring samples) – the 1305, 1315, 1325 results track Libby's theoretical line implying no enrichment or depletion, then 1335 shows a notable enrichment, 1345 and 1355 notable depletion.

Pearson (20 ring samples) – 1290-1310 steep enrichment; 1310-30 less enrichment; 1330-50 steep depletion

Interhemispheric (replicated 10-ring samples, two species) 1315-25 steep enrichment; 1325-35 enrichment switched off; 1335-45 and 1355 fairly steep depletion.

What may have been going on? Notice that this opposite behaviour and radio-carbon reversal seems to be earlier than the 1340s. In fact, if we look closely at the figures, we can postulate that the key changes begin somewhere between 1325 and 1335 with the long period of enrichment ending, and the curves changing direction towards depletion of radiocarbon. We could argue that the change takes place between 1335 and 1345 if we were to go solely with Stuiver's original 10-ring results, but then we find ourselves relying on a single radiocarbon date for the 1335 decade. Whereas, looking at the replicated northern/southern hemisphere data it is clear that the changes started between 1325 and 1335. So, let's go with the replicated data.

Looking again at *Figure 17* we see that from 1325-35 the slope of the various lines approximate to the slope of Libby's theory line. This implies that between these dates the system went from an enrichment mode, with excess radiocarbon being produced by incoming cosmic radiation, to a steady state mode where production of radiocarbon was balanced by decay of the isotope. It seems that from 1335-45 actual depletion clicks in, i.e. dilution of the radiocarbon in the atmosphere by the insertion of excess ^{12}C. This could either be by direct injection of some old radiocarbon-free carbon in relatively small quantities, or by the injection of quite a large amount of depleted carbon i.e. something that is a bit old as opposed to very old. The most likely source for depleted carbon is of course the oceans with relatively old water up-welling to the surface and exchanging with the atmosphere. An alternative possibility would have been to burn enormous areas of forest (in this case burning old trees will inject slightly old, slightly ^{14}C depleted carbon into the atmosphere). If we want to inject very old inert carbon it could come from burning coal/oil deposits or burning clathrate deposits or volcanoes or comets.

Figure 18 shows a possible interpretation of the radiocarbon turning point.[4] It is as if the curve was 'intending to continue enriching from 1325-35' (as indicated by the plain line in the figure) but it actually went into depletion. The heavy black arrow in the figure represents the difference between what we might have expected to happen and what actually happened. This difference is about 50 radiocarbon years but is only presented to give a feel for the nature of the change involved i.e. something slammed into reverse in a short period of time. The calibration curve is then noticeably static in 1335-55. This means that, at a first guess,

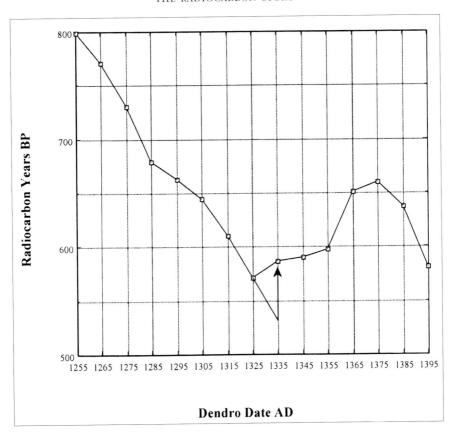

18 A simplified version of the mid-fourteenth century radiocarbon turning point based on the replicated data in *Figure 17. As originally published in* Dendrochronologia 20, 75

the sun was not doing anything very spectacular across the episode of the first wave of the Black Death. Yet, we have seen in Chapter 2 that the 1340s represent a global tree-ring growth downturn. If the sun was not changing this would imply that something else was controlling the reduction in tree growth! What? That is what we need to find out.

The reader could ask why scientists have not measured the radiocarbon activity in single year samples to get a clearer picture of these changes. The answer is all too simple. The calibration work was not aimed at answering this fourteenth-century question; it was aimed at looking at the radiocarbon offset between the northern and southern hemispheres over the last 1000 years. As is often the case in science we are piggy-backing on a piece of research which was actually done for some completely different reason. However, any way it is viewed, the radiocarbon calibration curve does show a major change in behaviour just in the run up to the Black Death. It should be apparent that the evidence is building up for something unusual taking place in the first half of the fourteenth century.

A BIT OF SERENDIPITY

Serendipity works well in science. Sometimes some obscure result has been published that appears to have no particular relevance to anything at the time of publication. Later circumstances may make the result important when it fits some new picture. This is what is about to happen with a study of CO_2 in air bubbles (trapped in south polar ice) now that we're asking questions about odd things happening in the middle of the fourteenth century. In the 1980s a team, including Hans Oeschger, were studying CO_2 in one of the South Pole ice cores. They noticed that there appeared to be an increase in the amount of CO_2 in the atmosphere about 700 years ago. In a speculative paper they pointed out the possibility that 'a cumulative input of about 45 GT C over the period AD 1200-1350' may have occurred.[5] Forty-five GT C simply means 45 gigatons (or 45 thousand million tons) of carbon. That's an awful lot of carbon. In fact the authors of the paper point out that it would represent 'about 6 per cent of the global pre-industrial

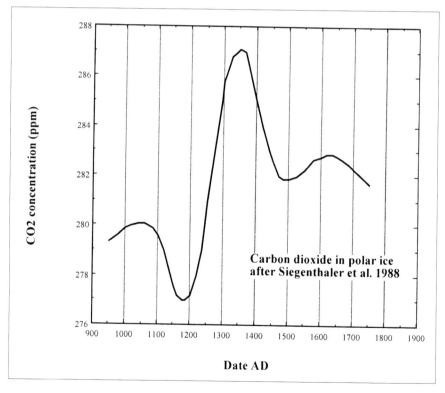

19 Suggested concentration of carbon dioxide in the atmosphere as deduced from an Antarctic ice core.[6] The elevated levels in the mid-fourteenth century beg the question of where the additional carbon dioxide came from. An ocean turnover event could be a possibility

live land biomass', i.e. 6 per cent of everything living on the surface of the planet. Since it seemed unlikely that this amount could have been burned off, they opted for:

> A possible net injection into the atmosphere of about 40 GT C of biospheric (perhaps oceanic) origin over the period AD 1250-1350.[7]

Now the nice thing about speculative research is that there is a bit of flexibility. The authors also mention that there is an uncertainty in the gas ages of about half a century (this is because, although the ice is well dated, the time when the gas was originally sealed in the ice is less well-dated). That flexibility leaves open the possibility that the massive injection of CO_2 may actually have been around the time – somewhere between 1330-50 – that the depletion occurs in the radiocarbon calibration curve. What the authors did not know, back in 1988 (but we now do know), is that the radiocarbon calibration curve shows continuous *enrichment* in the content of ^{14}C from about 1250 to about 1330 (see *Figures 16-18*). If the amount of radiocarbon in the atmosphere is enriching, i.e. increasing, no dilution with massive amounts of CO_2 can have taken place between these dates.

Therefore the dilution pretty certainly has to take place *after* 1330. *Figure 19* shows that the suggested atmospheric concentration of CO_2 increases around 1350. This would encourage the view of *a massive ocean turnover event of some kind taking place anywhere between 1330 and 1350*. As soon as this statement about 'ocean turnover between 1330 and 1350' is made, it throws up a recurring theme. Several writers at the time of the Black Death mention masses of dead fish:

> The waters of the ocean were drawn up as a vapour so corrupted by the multitude of dead and rotting fish that the sun was unable to consume it …. So it drifted away, an evil noxious mist, contaminating all it touched.[8]

> There have been masses of dead fish, animals and other things along the sea shore and in many places trees covered in dust … and all these things seem to have come from the great corruption of the air and earth.[9]

A massive injection of CO_2 implying an ocean turnover, when coupled with references to earthquakes and dead fish imply something very interesting going on in the run-up to 1350. It only remains to ask what could cause such a turnover event. Of course, research does not stand still. Recently further attempts have been made to refine the picture relating to past changes in the concentration of CO_2 in the atmosphere. These have looked at fresh ice-core results from Taylor Dome, Antarctica.[10] Additional studies have used the frequency of stomata on oak leaves to try to assess the past levels of CO_2.[11] However, none of this new information changes the basic proposition being made here. Namely, that the observed radiocarbon enrichment from 1250 to the 1330s is not compatible with increasing CO_2 in the atmosphere during that period. Increasing CO_2 is much more compatible with the *dilution of radiocarbon* which is seen after the 1330s and quite possibly just around 1350.

CONCLUSION

The radiocarbon calibration work is well known in scientific circles and its results are used on a daily basis by archaeologists worldwide. Details of the method are unlikely to have impinged much on the thinking of historians. The fact that the calibration was performed on precisely dated wood samples means that it has a high degree of chronological integrity and as such is pretty well compatible with other sources of historical data. Moreover, as with much of dendrochronology, the results are completely independent of past human activity; they can be used, therefore, to cast a fresh light on what was going on in one facet of the environment. Although it is not normal to think in this way: while human populations were going about their business in the fourteenth century, trees were recording the relative quality of their annual growth conditions, and sampling the amount of radiocarbon in the atmosphere. This is the 'history' that the trees recorded. The humans lived in the same environment and breathed the same atmosphere. They just failed to leave any systematic environmental record.

As we've now seen, elements of that same atmosphere were actually preserved in the ice cores as compressed bubbles of gas. Analysis of that gas is now giving us clues about some of the other things that were happening on the planet while humans were coughing their last and accepting that God was punishing them for their sins by sending the *pestilentia*. The precisely dated tree-ring chronologies underpinning the radiocarbon calibration provide the yardstick for assessing exactly when it was all happening.

4

THE AMERICAS

Although the story started with studies of European oak, in point of fact, dendrochronology has a much longer history in the United States. The sheer volume of results from the Americas means that it is worth taking a closer look at what records exist there, and what we can glean from them of relevance to the fourteenth century.

Dendrochronology was introduced, as a working method, in the American south-west. Andrew Douglass, an astronomer, was interested in extending records of tree growth back in time in the hope that they would elucidate solar cycles. His thinking was that in a semi-arid region one could expect the annual growth of trees to be controlled by available moisture. If that were the case, then *long-term trends* might provide a proxy record of changes in solar output. With this aim in mind, Douglass set out to extend the record of living pines in the region. He sought out archaeologists who were studying American pueblos, and ruins of the Anasazi, and used the ruins as a source of samples for tree-ring research. In this dry region, archaeologists were regularly finding beams in standing ruins and even charred timbers on destroyed sites. Gradually, across the 1920s, Douglass built up an understanding of the chronology of these Amerindian sites from as early as the eighth century.

As Douglass was piecing together his chronology he noticed that there were short runs of tree-ring pattern which were almost always present in particular periods. He called these *signature patterns*; for example, 'a set of four narrow rings followed by two wide rings with a noticeable narrow ring seven years later' occurred in the years 1215-27. If Douglass saw that particular pattern in a new piece of wood from a site he could immediately tell the date of those rings. Then all he had to do was count the rings forward to the outside of the sample and he could give the felling date. Douglass was very good at this. He memorised all the signature patterns in his chronologies so that he acted like a living tree-ring encyclopedia. Imagine being able to pick up a wood section, study the rings with a hand lens, recognise a signature pattern, count the rings to the bark surface and announce to the archaeologist that the tree had been felled in AD 1312! Douglass could sometimes do just that, demonstrating a really remarkable expertise.

To simplify the story, Douglass built a chronology back to 1284 and then had trouble linking this to a floating chronology that we now know spanned 701-1285. This is very analogous to the problem faced in Ireland across 1350. Eventually he found a timber that spanned 1380-1227 and bridged his 'gap' (it turned out that in fact a short overlap had existed between 1260 and 1285, but this had been too short to give a definitive link). This tree-ring bridge gave America, and the world, its first long year-by-year tree-ring chronology which immediately revolutionized the chronology of the American south-west. It also become clear that dendrochronology as a discipline was inherently important as a chronological and environmental indicator. The very act of building the chronology, and dating the Amerindian ruins, proved the potential of the method. It was this early success by Douglass that led ultimately to the growth of tree-ring research in Europe.

Before moving on, let us consider this original gap-bridging exercise a little further. Douglass set out to build a long chronology and that chronology turned out to have two easy bits, with lots of timbers, separated by a difficult bit, *the gap*. The gap took a lot of effort to bridge. Why? What was going on? Well it turns out that there is a glimmer of an answer to this question. Further research has shown that just where Douglass had that short overlap – from 1260-85 – there was a drought, a 'Great Drought'. In the 1970s Martin Rose and colleagues at Tucson undertook a detailed climate study based on tree-ring chronologies from Arroyo Hondo in New Mexico.[1] At this site, the ring patterns from fourteenth-century phases ran back across the thirteenth century. It turned out that, according to the trees, there was a great drought from 1276-99 which almost certainly made it impossible to sustain agriculture in the area. We can imagine people having to abandon settlements and possibly an increase in raiding for scarce food supplies. Certainly this was a period of stress. So, the very first 'tree-ring gap' in the world actually pointed a finger at a period of environmental stress. This was the first hint that gaps, although they just seem to be a nuisance to dendrochronologists, are usually indicating environmental problems of some nature. As we saw in Chapter 1, it was the Irish 'gap' in the mid-fourteenth century that gave rise to the interest in the period of the Black Death.

We can also use Arroyo Hondo as an example of what a detailed dendrochronological analysis can sometimes show. It demonstrates the power of dendrochronology when wood survives for dating, and for climatological analysis. Just a few details from the report will suffice to show what can be deduced. Rose and colleagues noted the drought episode from 1276-99, then went on to say:

Arroyo Hondo was established about AD 1300 when precipitation was increasing after a 50-year period of mostly below average values. It may be that by making desert farming possible ... the increased rainfall made this location attractive to settlers for the first time. Initially a small group of farmers constructed an alignment of rooms along the edge of the canyon.[2]

From the tree-ring response it was possible to deduce that rainfall remained above the long-term average for about the first 35 years of the fourteenth century. This in turn implies that agriculture was probably productive and population could expand. That is also implied by the archaeological findings:

> With ... favourable climatic conditions, the pueblo grew to nearly a hundred times its original size in the first three decades of the 1300s .... The settlement reached its greatest size around 1330, comprising 24 room blocks constructed around 10 ... enclosed plazas.[3]

So, the dendrochronologists were actually charting the whole development of this expanding site in real time and could infer the population density from the number of rooms as the construction grew. However, in the south-west conditions can turn marginal very quickly and, again, the combination of dendrochronology and dendroclimatology tell us what happened next:

> ... about AD 1335 the pattern of precipitation shifted toward high annual variability, with severe droughts separated by brief wet intervals ... soon after 1335 the town's population began to decline even more dramatically than it had increased...by about 1345 the pueblo was virtually abandoned (for the next 30 years) ....Then, sometime during the 1370s, a second phase of settlement began.[4]

It is sobering to think that in the years just before 1347, when the plague known as the Black Death arrived into Europe, changing environmental conditions in the American south-west were causing the abandonment of what were effectively agriculture-based towns. Two totally independent populations suffering at the same time, that does smack of a common cause. But, the only vector that can possibly be common between Europe and America at that time is climate change. That is if we ignore Fred Hoyle and Chandra Wickramasinghe's theory about diseases coming from space, and perhaps affecting the whole planet.[5] Readers will have noticed the proposed date of the turning point in the fortunes of the people of Arroyo Hondo was about 1335. We now know that this is not an arbitrary date; it is very close to the point where the radiocarbon calibration curve turns from enrichment to depletion (see Chapter 3).

THE LONGER AMERICAN CHRONOLOGIES

Before looking further at the archaeological chronologies that Douglass initiated, it is worth mentioning one or two other tree-ring applications that were sparked by him. Quite early on in his tree-ring work Douglass recognised the possibilities provided by some of the long-lived species in North America. For example, he put together a 3200-year chronology for giant sequoia (the giant redwoods of California) using sections from the stumps of these vast trees that were being logged in the early twentieth century. Douglass' successors then set out to look for even longer-lived trees and found the bristlecone pines that exist at high altitudes in Nevada and California. These trees can live for up to 5000 years. Moreover, when they die they tend not to rot, with the result that many ancient trees survive as fallen trunks. Using these living and dead trees, a number of Tucson-based dendrochronologists built suites of chronologies, the longest being around 8000 years and 5300 years in length. These were the trees used to provide the samples for the original Suess calibration that was mentioned in Chapter 3. One of the Tucson dendrochronologists, Val LaMarche, was keen to exploit the fact that, living at such high altitudes, bristlecone pines had to be sensitive to temperature in the growing season (in the same way as the Fennoscandian pines are temperature sensitive due to their growth in high latitudes). It was for this reason that quite a lot of chronologies were constructed for climatic-reconstruction purposes.

From the point of view of this chapter, the importance of the bristlecone pines is that we have a well-replicated set of chronologies. *Figure 20* shows nine bristlecone site chronologies, together with an average master chronology (made by simply adding the nine together) for the fourteenth century. What is immediately apparent is the dramatic reduction in ring width, in essentially all the chronologies, following the year 1333. This has to be related to a sudden reduction in temperature. Not only is there a sudden and dramatic decline in the bristlecone pines following 1333, but there is a 'switch' from an extended period of sustained positive (better than normal) growth from 1310-33, to a long period of below average growth from 1334-67. So, simply looking at this bristlecone record tells us a good deal about some dramatic, and extended, change affecting western North America immediately after 1333. Given that we have already looked at the radiocarbon calibration curve and identified a date close to 1335 as an effective turning point – from radiocarbon enrichment to depletion - this tends to reinforce the idea that there is an ocean component to this story. The consistency of this date with the story of Arroyo Hondo shows that at least some human populations in America were also affected by the changes.

It is interesting to see how different chronologies can contribute back-up to this set of observations. In the 1980s Louis Scuderi constructed another temperature-sensitive chronology from the upper tree line in the Sierra Nevada. This time he used foxtail pine and was able to produce a 2000-year temperature reconstruction.

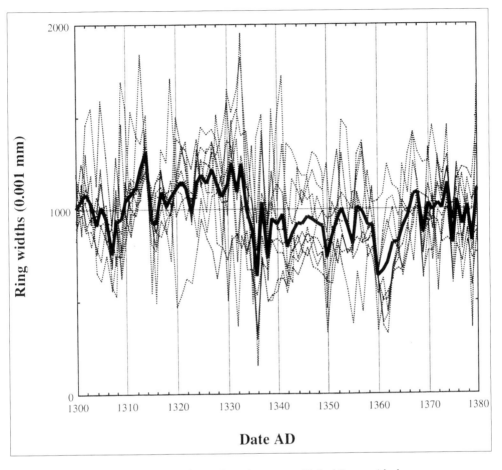

20 Nine bristlecone pine chronologies from the western United States with the average shown in bold. *Data courtesy Laboratory for Tree-Ring Research, University of Arizona at Tucson*

Of particular interest was his observation of several very cold years just around AD 540, a date we shall hear more of later. However, he listed other extreme years and some outstanding 20-year mean values. He observed that in his foxtail chronology the fifth-highest, positive, 20-year anomaly spanned 1314-33, with an excess temperature of 0.94 degrees centigrade.[6] Indeed, Ed Cook and Mike Edwards have also reported, again on the basis of tree-ring reconstructions, that 1338-47 was the second driest 10-year period in the last 800 years, in the south-western US.[7] This confirms the good-to-bad flip after 1333, observed in the bristlecone chronologies; it appears that in western America after 1333 it got both cooler and drier.

In the eastern United States dendrochronologists have used tree-rings to reconstruct river flow. Using a 950-year chronology from Arkansas they found that river flow was anomalous from 1330-46 and contains about six 'out of line' values in that short period. For example, 1330, 1334 and 1338 were all abnormally high, with the river-flow for 1341 being the highest value in the entire 950-year record.[8] In contrast, the 1342 and 1346 values were both anomalously low. This ties in well with Rose's statement, quoted earlier:

> … about AD 1335 the pattern of precipitation shifted toward high annual variability, with severe droughts separated by brief wet intervals …

Going back to the giant sequoia, these have been studied in order to deduce a drought record from low growth of the trees. At two sites, Camp Six and Giant Forest, researchers observed a severe drought in 1335; with no other between 1296 and 1351.[9] Putting these various strands together, after 1333 the climate experienced in North America was one of widespread variability, whether you were in the west, the south-west or the south-east. Something had clearly caused a shake up of the whole system.

Overall, it is quite clear that American tree-ring chronologies are a major resource which can provide various strands of both chronological and environmental information. As we saw in Chapter 1, accumulating archaeological tree-ring dates can provide information as well. If we go back to the archaeological chronologies, initiated by Douglass, and carried on by generations of his successors, we find an enormous archive of precise dates for archaeological remains. Since 1929, literally thousands of timbers have been dated in the south-west; from Arizona, New Mexico, Colorado and Utah. For example, in 1991 Robinson and Cameron could report on 27,000 dates from 1300 sites; an almost unimaginable amount of dating activity.[10] They listed their sites by earliest felling date on any site and also by latest felling date. The results are inherently interesting because they represent another one of those quasi-random samples of what is out there in the archaeological record. Remember, the archaeologists and dendrochronologists do not know the age of the sites when they are investigated; the dates only appear *after* tree-ring analysis. It is this 'randomness' factor that makes the distributions of such dates inherently powerful, i.e. they reflect real information. There is no 'theory' involved; it is an entirely empirical exercise.

Before presenting results from this massive dating survey, a few words are necessary about how these American dates were handled. Each site with a latest felling date in the fourteenth century was counted and its date noted. However, for sites with 'latest dates' after 1350 (i.e. sites whose latest dates can have no influence on the run-up to the Black Death period) any 'earliest dates' which fell between 1300 and 1350 were also noted. This may sound complicated but it is not. It is a very simple way of handling a robust set of dating results. So, the number of sites with felling dates was accumulated. *Figure 21* shows a raw plot of the number of sites, from the American south-west, across the fourteenth century.

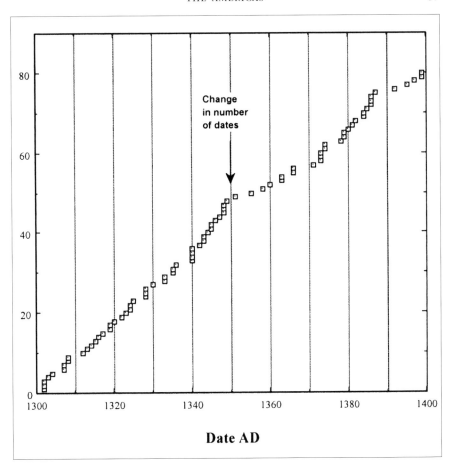

21 Running sum plot of the tree-ring dates for archaeological structures in the American south-west showing the turning point around AD 1350. *Data compiled by Bill Robinson and Catherine Cameron*

Here, on a continent supposedly not affected by the Black Death, in a large random sample we see a dramatic drop in the number of site dates after 1350. Just to spell this out, in the 1340s there are 16 dates, in the 1350s there are only 3. This has to be an interesting reflection of something negative (less felling activity providing less datable timbers in the record) going on in this part of the Americas at *exactly* the same time that the Black Death was inhibiting construction in Europe. Obviously there could be any number of environmentally related factors that could have caused this change in the rate of building activity. However, one cannot *a priori* rule out the arrival of some sort of 'plague'.

CONCLUSION

The American tree-ring records show that in the early fourteenth century there are good examples of site abandonment coincident with the run up to the Black Death. Indeed it is not possible to look at the similarity in dating between the Old and New Worlds without wondering if the 'plague' actually got to America. Remember if we start to think like this we would have to also wonder just what the plague was. The Old and New Worlds were supposed to be isolated from one another in the fourteenth century. If both these areas were affected by 'plague' then it probably was not bubonic plague (as people have been saying with increasing clamour for some time) and one might have to start wondering about concepts such as environmental causes of disease, or even diseases from space (disease in the broad sense of 'something from space that kills people'). We shall come back to both the date and the issue of Hoyle and Wickramasinghe's ideas later.

It so happens, that Stuiver's radiocarbon results (Chapter 3) across this period were on wood from the western United States, proximate to the Pacific Ocean. Referring back to *Figure 20*, the bristlecone pines show that dramatic reduction in ring width starting just after 1333. It may well be that this is a physical reflection of something affecting the Pacific Ocean which in turn may be a part reason for the change in ^{14}C in Stuiver's calibration results. One gets a feeling that a joined-up environmental picture is beginning to emerge.

5

DESCRIPTIVE MYTH

By now the reader has hopefully got the general idea of what this story is about. We do not have all that good a grasp on just what went on, even in the relatively recent past. It is probably fair to say that what we do not know outweighs what we do know. This is not how most people view the issue. It seems to be widely assumed that we (scientists and historians) *know* about the past in some detail. Nothing could be further from the truth. So, this chapter is going to re-tell the story of how the tree-ring chronologies led to the finding of a series of, what appear to be, profound environmental events which took place in the last several millennia. This is all part of building up a feeling for how tree-rings impart information. It may seem like a digression but hopefully it will all make sense later. Readers should note that one of the tree-ring events, at AD 540, coincides remarkably with the start of the great plague at the time of Justinian. This coincidence will be expanded upon in Chapter 6.

Back in the mid-1980s, interrogation of the ring patterns that made up the 7400-year Irish oak chronology turned up a series of 'narrowest ring' events at 3195, 2345, 1628, 1159, 207 BC and AD 540.[1] These were points in time when numbers of oak trees growing on different Irish peat bogs, simultaneously exhibited the worst growth – the *narrowest ring widths* – in their long lives. It was evident from this widespread occurrence of poor growth conditions in Irish oaks, that these events were pretty certainly *catastrophically* bad. Ireland is, after all, a small temperate island; its inhabitants are not used to extremes of climate, nor, in recent times, are its oaks. From the start, when these ancient, narrowest-ring events were uncovered in the data, there was a strong presumption that the events were caused by the loading of the atmosphere with dust and gas from major explosive eruptions. This was because in one of the earliest Greenland ice-core records there were layers of volcanic acid at dates that coincided fairly well with the dates of the narrowest ring events.

The problem was that several lines of reasoning actually suggested that the volcano hypothesis did not make that much sense. For example, the events in the trees tended to last for longer than volcanologists were comfortable with. The volcanic material, even from a big explosive eruption, is not injected all that high into the stratosphere; thus over just a few years it should rain out. A general consensus, from people who study volcanoes and their effects, would be that the worst consequences of a big explosive eruption should be over in about three years. For example, Mt Pinatubo that erupted in 1991 did cause some global cooling over about two years. Why, if the effects of volcanoes only last for a few years, did the tree-ring events last for most of a decade (3199-90 BC; 2354-45 BC; 1628-23 BC and AD 536-45), even two decades in the case of 1159-41 BC? Obviously one answer to that conundrum could be that the trees' response to the initial trigger event was longer than the duration of the environmental event itself. While this was always a possibility, it was only that, a possibility. There was the alternative possibility that the duration of the events was indeed longer than three years. This is the classic dilemma for the scientist, several possible explanations and no easy way to work out which one is correct.

Another problem with the issue of volcanoes and severe environmental events is that, over time, there are quite a lot of them; big volcanoes erupt pretty regularly. Take the last two centuries. In 1815 there was the eruption of Tambora in Indonesia. This was classed as one of the most explosive eruptions in the last 10,000 years. However, it had only moderate environmental effects on a global scale. It did not cause the collapse of any civilizations or indeed anything of that nature. It did provide a poor summer or two in the North Atlantic. Then there was Krakatau in 1883, again no real repercussions; same with Katmai (1912), Agung (1962) and, as we've seen, Pinatubo in 1991. It does look as if the sorts of volcanoes that have been erupting in the last 10,000 years do not cause truly *catastrophic* environmental events. Why then should we observe only a small number of these long-duration, narrowest-ring, events in Irish oaks?

To this discussion we could add the fundamental problem with the early ice-core dating of the acid layers in Greenland. The errors on the first ice-core dates tended to be of the order of 30-100 years. This meant that the *apparent* association of the narrowest rings, in the precisely dated tree-ring chronologies, with the ice acidities was based on a weak comparison. The date ranges for the layers of volcanic acid could be from decades to centuries wide; it had probably been unwise to make the comparison in the first place. All in all, while the volcano hypothesis maintained the current paradigm – that volcanoes cause cooling and climate upset – in fact the evidence of the extreme tree-ring events actually suggested that volcanoes should not do that.

In this vein, one particularly interesting piece of evidence that weakened the idea of volcanoes causing 'long-drawn-out' environmental downturns related to sulphur. The conventional wisdom is that explosive volcanoes inject sulphur high into the stratosphere. There it is rapidly converted to droplets of sulphuric acid which are (allegedly) very good at reflecting back sunlight and causing cooling at the earth's surface. The problem was, and is, that some of the biggest sulphur layers in the ice cores were not associated with any obvious response in the tree-rings. A good example is the 1258/9 sulphur layer that occurs in the ice in both Greenland and the Antarctic. It does not seem to be directly associated with any long-drawn-out environmental consequences. The same could be said for the big acid layer in the AD 930s. There is no obvious response in tree-ring chronologies.[2] There are other examples of the same thing. Overall, during the 1990s the hypothesis – that ordinary explosive volcanoes could cause the extreme events seen in the tree rings – existed; however, it was not in any way proven, and, as outlined, the hypothesis suffered from a variety of problems.

Thus, it was not all that much of a surprise when, around 1993, it materialized that the most recent, and chronologically constrained, narrowest-ring event – that at AD 540 – did not coincide with any well-dated layer of volcanic acid in the Greenland ice. Let's just set this issue out in a little detail, because it is important. Back in 1993 there were only four published ice-core records relating to volcanoes. When these were looked at, it was found that there was no good evidence for a major, environmentally effective, volcanic eruption anywhere in the time window 536-45.[3] The four ice cores were Crête (which stopped at around AD 550),[4] Camp Century (which was not analysed across the last two millennia),[5] Dye3 (which in an initial analysis had a major acid spike at 540+/-10, but which subsequently had the date revised)[6] and GISP2 (which had 14m of core 'trashed' between c.AD 614 and c.AD 545).[7] It is now known, on the basis of three replicated ice cores (the three European cores, Dye3, GRIP and NGRIP), that there is no significant volcanic-acid signal in the time window 536-45.[8] The latest statement from the ice-core workers says specifically:

> With the chemistry and the isotope data it is possible to do a very precise dating for the eruption. The volcanic eruption is dated to AD 527 +/- 1 year. The AD 527 volcanic eruption is the only eruption in the period.[9]

The authors go on to say that this AD 527 volcano is the only likely candidate to have caused the 536-45 global event, but that the dating 'suggest(s) that the event is not the same one described by other sources'.

The 1993 realization that there was no *good* evidence for a major, environmentally effective, volcano around 540, then allowed the posing of the next logical question – 'if the 540 event was not caused by a volcano, what is the next most likely cause of a global environmental downturn?' The answer to that question was pretty unequivocal. The next most likely cause of a global environmental downturn, as witnessed in a suite of tree-ring chronologies from around the world (from Mongolia, Siberia, Fennoscandia, Europe, North and South America) had to be loading of the atmosphere from space. Inevitably, once that spectre was raised, comets, or comet debris, entered the realm of consideration.

So, from the mid-1990s, consideration was being given to the possibility that the 540 environmental event might have been caused by some interaction with a comet or its debris.

To be frank, despite quite explicit publication relevant to this subject, the issue has been roundly ignored.[10] Worse still, in 1999 the journalist David Keys published his book *Catastrophe*[11] in which he came out with the idea that a super-volcano had erupted on the site of Krakatau in February 535. Now, while there was not a shred of realistic evidence for this suggestion, the publicity associated with his book ensured that the 'idea' of a 535 super-volcano developed overnight into a 'fact'. For example, it is included as a fact in innumerable timelines on the Internet. But it is not a fact, and its endless repetition will not make it a fact. It would seem more sensible to believe the ice-core workers who have replicated scientific evidence relevant to the question and, as quoted above, they are unequiv-ocal on the issue. Keys' hypothetical super-volcano cannot be reconciled in any way with the statements of the ice-core community (not least because the effects of a super-volcano would *undoubtedly* have been recognised by geologists and others).

It is important to get the order of this debate correct. The suggestion that the AD 540 event might have been caused by a comet was based purely on (i) the recognition of the event in tree-ring chronologies from around the world, and (ii) the lack of any clear volcanic signal in the, now well-dated, Greenland ice record. This was a purely scientific question and required no use of historical infor-mation. What was not realized until around 1995 was the fact that three British astrophysicists, Mark Bailey, Victor Clube and Bill Napier, had proposed in 1990 that, in their view (based on the incidence of large meteor showers), the earth was at risk of bombardment by comet debris in the time window 400-600.[12] Nor was it realized that the issue of what happened around 540 would give rise to a whole book,[13] in fact two books,[14] dealing with mythology associated with the 540 event. These considerations, and growing accumulations of information relevant to each of the event dates, meant that by the early 2000s it was becoming clear that all the narrowest-ring events seemed to stand a chance of being extra-terrestrial in origin.[15]

It is worth mentioning that throughout the period since the publication of those narrowest-ring dates in 1988, the most intriguing point had to be that the dates just *would not* go away. More and more information kept coming in to give the distinct impression that these dates actually represented turning points in human history. Without going into too much detail (because the detail is pub-lished elsewhere and can be followed up from the references if desired) let's take a brief look at the dates of the several tree-ring events, to give a flavour for anyone not familiar with the issues.

3195 BC

This date marks a distinct interruption in the middle of the Neolithic period in Ireland and Britain. The later Neolithic is different from the preceding early Neolithic. Two tree-ring chronologies, from low-lying areas in the east and west of England, both start within a decade of this date. In the Near East this date pretty much marks the start of literate civilization. There are anomalous levels of sulphate in the ice cores in the early 3100s BC and these have been interpreted as ocean-derived rather than volcanic.[16] There are even hints of alterations in wind direction wherein a lake dwelling in Switzerland shows a change of house orientation at 3204 BC (the sites are dated by dendrochronology which allows this degree of precision).[17] Overall, 3200 BC is not an arbitrary date, it seems to be a major turning point of some sort. Of at least anecdotal interest, Ötzi, the prehistoric man uncovered in the Alps has been suggested to date to around this same period.[18] Given that he had been frozen continuously for around 5300 years, it suggests something unusual about the circumstances of his original preservation. Several of the factors (e.g. the coastal location of the English oak chronologies, the oceanic sulphate and the Swiss change of wind direction) all hint at something affecting the oceans 5200 years ago.

2345 BC

This event starts in the Irish oaks in 2354 BC and lasts until at least 2345. This is as good a date as any for the end of the Neolithic and the start of the Bronze Age in the British Isles – a major cultural change separating the age of stone-using agriculturalists from the first metal users. It is not far from the generally accepted date for a major collapse of civilization in the Near East.[19] But the most surprising thing was the discovery that it represented a 'known' date in ancient legend/history/myth. For example, it includes the date given by Archbishop Ussher for the biblical Flood (2349). It is the traditional date for the *first* emperor in China, Yao, who is famous for the *huge floods* that 'overtopped the mountains' in his reign. It is also a traditional date for an occasion when the same first emperor met the Divine Archer, Shên I, who saved the earth from the 10 suns that were threatening the planet (the first emperor is traditionally dated to 2357 and he meets the Divine Archer in 2346).[20] Surprisingly, in the earliest section of the *Irish Annals*, compiled in the seventeenth century from ancient sources, it is recorded that around this time:

> 2341 BC In this year overflowed Lake Arbreath and Lake Annim in Midia.[21]

Overall, the strange connection of three separate stories involving calamities around 2350 BC does suggest that something happened that was remembered as a 'time since when', i.e. a *time from which years were counted*. Surprisingly (or perhaps not so surprisingly), Ussher's date for the Flood was accepted by both Isaac Newton, and Edmond Halley, who both believed that a comet on a 575-year orbit was responsible for the catastrophe.[22]

1628 BC

This date first came to notice as a frost-ring event in 1627 BC in LaMarche's bristlecone pine record, but subsequently showed up, starting in 1628, in Irish oaks. Intriguingly, the *Irish Annals* also have an entry around this time, remarkably similar to the entry for 2341 BC:

> 1629 BC Eruption of these nine lakes ... (followed by a list of the nine lakes).[23]

Since its discovery by LaMarche, the 1628 BC event has been recognised as a global event, probably involved in the collapse of the Hsia dynasty in China (and its replacement by the Shang dynasty), and marking the disturbed Second Intermediate Period in Egypt. Chinese records from the time (unfortunately not precisely dated, i.e. they relate to the dynastic change but do not give an exact calendar year) refer to the sun being dim, frosts in the summer, famines and widespread fatalities. One relevant story also refers to two 'suns' being in the sky; one in the east and one in the west. The last Hsia king, Chieh, is credited with saying 'When that sun dies, you and I, we shall all perish'.[24] This is a fitting end for a dynasty, when heaven withdraws its mandate from the emperor and his dynasty. What better cause than a comet – a second sun – 'setting' and giving rise to an environmental disaster. Logic would suggest that one of the 'suns' had to be a close comet as bright as the sun.

For many years it was argued, not least by this author, that the driving force behind this environmental downturn was the eruption of Santorini in the Aegean. The arguments about the exact date of this massive volcanic eruption have now gone on for more than 20 years. Currently the scientific consensus is that the eruption actually took place in the 1640s, and had relatively little environmental effect.[25] This is consistent with the general downgrading of the effects of volcanoes mentioned above. If this is true, it leaves us with a major unexplained environmental event following 1628 BC. Unexplained, that is, unless we take account of the Chinese 'second sun', the sun being dim, the summer frosts and the famines.

1159 BC

This event lasts from 1159-1141 BC and falls at a particularly interesting point in history. The twelfth century marks the collapse of civilization in the Mediterranean and the beginning of the four-century-long Greek Dark Ages. It also marks the end of the important Shang dynasty in China. It has to be a possibility – given the vagaries of dating this far back in time – that these two events actually took place at the same time; right in the middle of the twelfth century.

Here it is worth mentioning the myths associated with the end of the Shang dynasty in the twelfth century BC. At the defeat of the evil King Chóu (traditionally in 1122 BC but let's just say 'around the twelfth century BC'), there is a mythical 'Battle of Mu' when sky entities (spirits/immortals/gods) and earthly armies are doing battle. In the west, the Battle of Troy also involves sky gods and earthly armies. Given that any battle with both gods and men is most likely mythical in character, it would seem appropriate to believe that both 'mythologies' were describing the same thing. That sort of consideration immediately implies that, if they are describing the same thing, they were probably witnessing the battles in the sky. If that was the case then the most likely date would lie in the mid-twelfth century.

The dilemma of course is that while the tree-rings and the ice cores are purely scientific endeavours, almost no one in the modern science (or indeed art or history) community is geared up to cope with mythology. Mythology is, to all intents and purposes, not allowable in scientific or historical discussion. However, as a chronologist, it seems reasonable to note that these myths, for some reason, come with dates, and these dates seems to stand up to quite a reasonable degree of comparison with real events evidenced in the tree-ring chronologies. To consolidate the idea that catastrophic events seem to attract mythologies, here is an additional mythical story. It makes an important linkage that essentially proves that these stories contain real information.

As mentioned above, by tradition there is a Chinese Divine Archer who saves the earth from the threat of 10 suns in the year 2346 BC. That is the year when the emperor Yao meets a man carrying a bow wrapped in 'red stuff'. The incredible ability of this archer causes the emperor to christen him 'the Divine Archer' (Shén I). At this time there were terrible catastrophes which included 10 suns in the sky, famines, floods etc. The Divine Archer set out to seek the cause of these catastrophic events and found that they were due to the activities of one Fei Lien (a wind spirit).[26] So far so good, we have one story which has a date synchronous with one of our tree-ring events around 2350 BC. But, in the stories Fei Lien – who was responsible for the calamities in the twenty-fourth century BC – was also a minister of King Chóu, the last emperor of the Shang.[27] So, someone in China recognised the similarity between what happened in the twenty-fourth century BC and what happened in the twelfth century.

This can only be explained by people in the twelfth century having access to records of what had happened in the twenty-fourth century BC and recognising the same 'entity'. The logic has to be that in both cases they recognised something in the sky. Bizarrely, given this hint that the battles of Mu and Troy might just relate to the same sky event, the most famous mythical battle in Irish tradition – the Battle of Moytura – can also be linked to the same event. This is because there is one ancient Irish anecdote that says that the Battle of Moytura was at the same time as the Battle of Troy.[28] Again, the Battle of Moytura is peopled by sky gods including the great Celtic god Lugh who is described in one text as 'coming up in the west, as bright as the sun, and with a long arm', i.e. a comet god.

Now one can understand many readers throwing up their hands, or their heads, and thinking 'this is the lunatic fringe'. A few years ago this would have been a reasonable attitude. But now there is sufficient evidence linking *dated* myths and *dated* tree-ring events to make the quite plausible argument that some of the myths do contain a core of truth. For example, it is almost certainly no accident that the traditional date for the Flood (2349 BC) coincides with one tree-ring event which spans 2354-45 BC, *and* coincides with a traditional date for Chinese catastrophes at 2346 BC, *which is then linked* to another tree-ring event at 1150 BC. So, just to reinforce the idea that some of these mythical stories may hold a core of truth, here is another one.

This story is set in the AD 670s, during the Tang dynasty. A character, Liu I, features in a complicated love story wherein he meets the daughter of the Dragon king (the Dragon king is a Lord of Heaven) and takes a letter from her to the Dragon king's palace. The description of the palace – set in a 'lake', with columns of white quartz, curtains of crystal and jewelled ceiling – is clearly a description of the sky. In the palace Liu I met with the Dragon king, Ling Hsü, and the Dragon king's brother Ch'ien T'ang. Liu I asks the Dragon king about his brother. The Dragon king's reply is interesting:

> He (Ch'ien T'ang) is so wild and impetuous that I am afraid he might do great damage. The great flood which covered the earth for nine years during the reign of the emperor Yao was caused by him in his anger. Because he had a quarrel with a heavenly ruler he caused a great flood which reached to the summits of the five tall mountains.[29]

The reader cannot be expected to experience this author's excitement when this Chinese folktale turned up. The Irish tree-rings show a severe environmental event lasting for a decade from 2354 BC down to 2345 BC. It involves what looks like an inundation of Lough Neagh, the largest lake in Ireland and Britain. Here is a Chinese folktale describing the entity that caused the *nine years of floods* at the time of Yao (the tale names Yao specifically so there is no doubt about which flood is being described; Yao's traditional date of accession is 2357 BC). The entity is Ch'ien T'ang and he lives in the sky. The story then describes Ch'ien T'ang in more detail:

… a sudden uproar broke out, a noise rending the sky and shaking the earth and causing the whole palace (the sky) to tremble, and causing smoke and clouds to billow out with a fierce hissing. A red dragon burst in (Ch'ien T'ang) a thousand feet long, with flashing eyes, a blood red tongue, scarlet scales and a fiery beard. The column to which he had been fettered was dragged along by him on a chain through the air. Snow, rain and hail were swirling in wild confusion. There was a thunderclap and the dragon soared up towards the sky and disappeared.[30]

We shall see that the description of the sky entity that caused the flood at the time of Yao bears a passable description of a Tunguska-class fireball (Tunguska was a *c.*15-megaton airburst that took place after a fireball traversed the sky over Siberia on June 30 1908; see Chapter 7). But the story does not end there. The Dragon king's brother has flown away to punish the evildoers who had treated his niece rather badly. When he returns he is asked what he did. The conversation in the story goes thus:

Ch'ien T'ang: I fought those damned dragons and utterly defeated them.
The Dragon king: How many did you kill?
Ch'ien T'ang: Six hundred thousand.
The Dragon king: Was farmland damaged?
Ch'ien T'ang: Over some eight hundred miles.

This is very specific information. We know that at Tunguska, in 1908, an area of approximately 2000km² of Siberian forest was flattened by the 15-megaton airburst. Now we see a Chinese story from the 670s where the sky entity, who was responsible for the floods around 2350 BC, and who was also present in the twelfth century BC, could damage 'eight hundred miles of farmland'. There is not much doubt that these stories preserve a memory of dated catastrophic events wherein pieces of space debris (probably fragments of comets) entered the earth's atmosphere at high velocity and exploded with catastrophic results on the ground. Oh yes, for anyone interested, the Dragon king's daughter marries Liu I and they live together for 10,000 thousand years which is pretty close to 'happily ever after'.

It is apparent that these stories are not 'made up'. They contain real information, often quite specific in character, and frequently they come with dates, that only now, with the advent of tree-ring chronologies, make sense. It is particularly interesting that the people who translated these Chinese stories did so many years before tree-rings made it possible to understand the significance of some of the traditional dates. Clearly, it is time for specialist scholars to go back to the original texts, in Chinese, and re-translate them knowing now what sorts of events they are actually describing. We have to remember that the original translators can have had little idea that these stories contained real information, they just did the best they could to translate them faithfully as fairy stories or folktales.

CONCLUSION

Although there is not space in this book to develop the mythical theme further, it should already be clear that myths should not be ignored. The fact that they come with dates which link separate events, makes it impossible that these are meaningless 'made up' stories. The additional fact, that each of the Irish 'narrowest-ring events' relates to pre-existing dated stories, reinforces the idea that it was the same environmental events that affected the Irish trees that caused the problems and dynastic changes around the Old World.

We have to think of what this means in the correct light. In the distant past, people did not necessarily compose straight descriptive text. Rather, they produced 'stories' that were originally oral. In a recent book on mythology, Barber and Barber have pointed out that in pre-literate societies information had to be compressed for purposes of transmission.[31] They suggest that the key points were 'encoded' in such a way that story-tellers could decompress them, and re-embellish the tale. They show that in one extreme case a story had been handed down for some 7000 years by native peoples living in the vicinity of Crater Lake, Oregon. These people had a taboo on going near the circular lake which was bound up with a story of an angry god who lived under a mountain and who caused the mountain to erupt. We now know that mountain as the volcano, Mount Mazama, which erupted around 7000 years ago, leaving the collapsed caldera that is now filled with Crater Lake. Barber and Barber conclude that myths have a core of truth; it is just that in many cases we do not (yet) know how to understand them. In the next chapter this theme will be developed to show that, apart from myths preserving truthful cores, there has also been extensive use of metaphor in the recording of past events. Sometimes it is only by taking account of both myths and metaphors that some important past events can be properly understood.

This is also the place to explain the direction this text is taking. This chapter has attempted to demonstrate that some dated information from the distant past – that at first acquaintance seems nonsensical (i.e. myth) – can actually be interpreted in a quite rational way. The Black Death of the fourteenth century sits essentially halfway between the modern 'rational' world and the sixth century which falls into this earlier 'mythical' world. All modern scholarship tries to understand the Black Death in a modern clinical paradigm. Any statements from the fourteenth century that sound 'odd' or 'mythical' or 'irrational' are ruthlessly pared away and ignored. Yet it is very clear that the earlier mythical stories cited in this chapter, irrespective of when they were written down, contain a pretty clear memory of specific ancient happenings of a catastrophic character. The hint is that we should not dismiss the odd stories relating to the fourteenth-century catastrophe out of hand.

6

DESCRIPTIVE METAPHOR

The reader has now been exposed to the novel idea that some of the best and most relevant records about past catastrophic events are preserved in dated myths and tree rings. In this chapter the concept can be extended to show that, in the case of the latest of the narrowest-ring events, namely the AD 540 catastrophic event, a number of contemporary writers used biblical metaphor to leave descriptions of what happened. This discovery came as a surprise because one does not expect hidden messages from the past. However, the fact that they exist has interesting implications for the way some information is conveyed. It is very much in line with the tone of Barber and Barber that the difficulty lies in our inability to understand the messages that have been left in myth (and now metaphor). This chapter is rather long but its importance lies in a new understanding of how some ancient writing may need to be handled. If apparently strange statements (and the reader will undoubtedly be struck by just how strange some of the metaphors are) were both accurate and directly relevant in the sixth century, why should the same not apply to apparently strange statements in the fourteenth century?

To understand just how bizarre this notion is, it is necessary to take a closer look at the whole 536-45 package. Perhaps the place to start is with the normally accepted view. In the same way that the Black Death has mostly been regarded as bubonic plague, so the plague at the time of Justinian is often treated as an earlier outbreak of the same disease. Typically writers devote just a few lines to this earlier plague, stating that it arrived into Constantinople in 542. Of course, most writers on the subject have not been aware of the tree-ring evidence for a complex, global, environmental downturn spanning this same period. The existence of this downturn completely changes the issue of the plague and indeed raises questions as to what the plague actually was. As noted in the last chapter, the comet-cause scenario for the 540 event opens up previously unconsidered possibilities.

GETTING INTO THE MINDSET

When the 540 event was first recognised to be global in character it was sup-posed, due to the work of Stothers and Rampino, that the happening at 536-7 was volcanic.[1] This was because of records of a severe 'dry fog', or dim sun, at that time. They noted a comment by the sixth-century Byzantine author Procopius:

> During this year a most dread portent took place. For the sun gave forth its light without brightness … and it seemed exceedingly like the sun in eclipse, for the beams it shed were not clear.[2]

And another by John Lydus:

> The sun became dim … for nearly the whole year … so that the fruits were killed at an unseasonable time.[3]

Reports from Constantinople suggested climatic upset for more than a year and a late chronicler, Michael the Syrian, apparently elaborated that:

> The sun became dark and its darkness lasted for eighteen months. Each day it shone for about four hours, and still this light was only a feeble shadow … the fruits did not ripen and the wine tasted like sour grapes.[4]

A contemporary Italian record by Cassiodorus states:

> The sun … seems to have lost its wonted light, and appears of a bluish colour. We marvel to see no shadows of our bodies at noon, to feel the mighty vigour of the sun's heat wasted into feebleness, and the phenomena which accompany an eclipse prolonged through almost a whole year. We have had … a summer without heat … the crops have been chilled by north winds … the rain is denied….[5]

These quotations make it clear that something unusual had happened and, on the basis of the descriptions, Stothers suggested that this was the most effective dust-veil in the last two millennia.[6] However, we can note that the references are focussed down onto 536/537. Yet, the tree-rings suggest two separate components of the event, one in 536 and another 'around 540', see *Figure 22*. Historically the plague at the time of Justinian is believed to have started as early as 540 and to have definitely arrived into Constantinople in 542. For the purposes of discussion, we will take it that the comet hypothesis is correct, i.e. the 540 event was caused, one way or another, by a comet or its debris. Interestingly, even though history books do not tell us overtly about a brush with a comet, there are several references to comets just around 540. For example, Gibbon mentions a 'great comet' in 539 that 'caused worry of calamitous things to come' and whose 'prognostications were abundantly fulfilled'.[7] The medieval historian, Roger of Wendover, writing in the thirteenth century, makes the following statement concerning 540/541: '540 Battles in the Air'. The reference is probably to aurorae seen in France [Britton's suggestion]. Roger of Wendover has an account of this:

> In the year of grace 541, there appeared a comet in Gaul, so vast that the whole sky seemed on fire. In the same year there dropped real blood from the clouds … and a dreadful mortality ensued ….[8]

With these references to comets around 540 we might assume that historians were well aware of a comet-based environmental event around 540. Nothing could be further from the truth. No historian refers to such a thing. In fact, when this came up as an issue in a review of Keys' book, *Catastrophe*, the comment by Roger of Wendover was dismissed as 'medieval fantasy' apparently because it was uncorroborated.[9] In fact it is now corroborated, in the sense that a plausible, independent, hypothesis (based on a global tree-ring downturn) exists suggesting that the earth's atmosphere was loaded by comet debris around 540. We shall see later that there is further corroborative evidence for the extraterrestrial hypothesis. (Indeed, in passing, it is worth mentioning another uncorroborated event from around the same time. Walford, in his collation of past events, mentions 'an earthquake, the effects of which are believed to have been felt over nearly the whole world' in 543.[10] Later, we shall see that this comment may also make some sense.)

That is enough background for the purposes of this chapter. Let us, for the sake of discussion, take it that the earth did indeed have a brush with debris from a comet around AD 540. Pieces of comet exploding in the upper atmosphere caused a dust-veil which, in turn, caused a severe environmental downturn that affected trees, food supply and humans. The reader has already been introduced at some length to the idea that myth can contain real information – the Chinese stories relating to the time of Yao being a case in point. So it should not now be a surprise that the time window 536-45 contains the myth of the death of King Arthur. Arthur, despite constant attempts to turn him into a warrior king is undoubtedly a Celtic god. He comes from the same group of Celtic deities as Cúchulainn, Lugh, Mongan and Finn, and it can reasonably be argued that all of these are comet gods.[11] Lugh, in particular, is described in one story as 'being as bright as the sun, coming up in the west, and having a long arm'. Given that he is without doubt a sky god, what else can come up in the west, as bright as the sun, having a long arm, other than a comet?

Now, people who may be willing to believe that there is a core of truth in Chinese myths may have more difficulty stomaching Arthur as a comet. So, here is a short story that makes the essential point.

If we turn to Turner's *Anglo Saxons*, we find a nineteenth-century view of Arthur. Turner says 'His sister Anna married Llew, brother of the famous Urien …

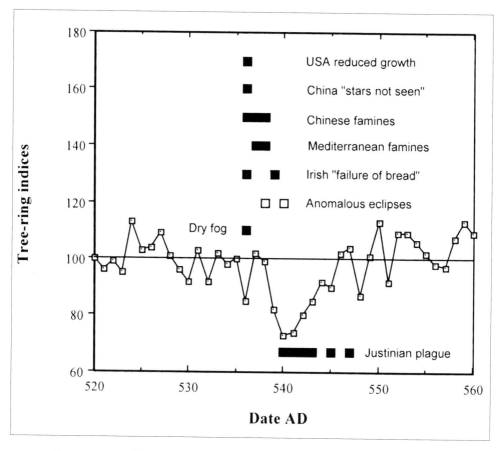

22 The 540 event as first published in *The Holocene* in 1994. The environmental effects on tree-rings serve to link the events of 536 to the outbreak of plague after 540

Medrawd was her son'.[12] So, Arthur's brother-in-law is Llew (the Welsh version of Lugh) who in turn is the brother of Urien. With that lineage, we should not be surprised at the descriptive elements used by Taliesin (Merlin) in describing Urien:

> Urien, the chief of Reged, has been most extolled. He was the son of Cynvarc the Aged. Taliesin has addressed to him several poems, with warm panegyric .... In these he calls him the head of the people; the shield of warriors; the most generous of men; bounteous as the sea; the thunderbolt of Cymry. He compares his onset to the rushing of the waves; and to the fiery meteors moving across the heavens.[13]

Given that it has already been proposed that Arthur was a comet, and that around AD 540 pieces of comet were striking the atmosphere, we can now note, not just the fact that in this story Arthur's brother-in-law is the comet god Lugh, but

Lugh's brother Urien has 'thunderbolt' and 'fiery meteor' imagery. Urien gives us other links. It is widely held that it is Morgan who is Arthur's sister; she is well known as Morgan le Fay (Anna, Morgana, Morgan, the names are interchangeable) who is one of nine fays 'skilled in flying swiftly through the air and in the art of healing' who live in Avalon. In one story:

> Morgan is married to King Urien of Gorre. The name of his country … suggests the other-world, the Ile de Voirre or Isle of Glass.[14]

So not only does Morgan live in Avalon – the otherworld – she is married to the King of the Isle of Glass, i.e. the king of the otherworld. As the Glass Castle is a metaphor for the sky, and as the wounded Arthur is taken to the Glass Castle on Avalon, it stands to reason that he was in the sky. This is just one example of many concerning Arthur's sky credentials. It is worth mentioning in this regard the widespread belief that he is not dead, but will some day return. It is possible to go on like this endlessly. For example, one well-known Arthurian motif is 'the Wasteland' caused by the 'Dolorous Blow' that destroys three kingdoms. Given Arthur's death date one could be forgiven for wondering where these concepts came from if they *were not* triggered by a catastrophic environmental event.

It seems that specifying a global environmental event spanning AD 536-45 immediately opens up another chapter of myth. Put simply, a comet sky god just happens to die at the event. This is more than the history books tell us, although both Gibbon and Roger of Wendover got pretty close! But notice that we have just seen the metaphorical use of 'Glass Castle' for 'the sky'. For some reason – and it is not altogether clear what the reason was – just around this 540 period there is widespread use of metaphor in contemporary writings. In this case the documents are not myths but mainstream historical documents accepted as credible sources (but not previously fully understood). There are two issues that arise at this point and they relate to the attitude of the Church on the one hand and to mythology on the other. It does not much matter in what order these issues are handled but as will become clear they dovetail quite well. The attitude of the Church seemed best summed up by a throw-away line in Bower's *History of the Popes*, published in 1750. Bower was a scholar and a member of the Inquisition (whatever that may mean by the eighteenth century). In his history, which runs right across the 540 period, he says the following:

> 539 The following year 540 nothing happened worthy of notice.[15]

This has to be a significant comment because there are other years in the sixth century where he provides no information, but it is only 539/540 that he 'highlights' with this peculiarly negative comment. So, a member of the Inquisition researching the history of the papacy felt moved to tell us quite specifically that nothing happened in a year when trees around the world were experiencing aspects of the worst environmental event in the last two millennia.

This may seem like labouring a fairly minor point (a single sentence in an eighteenth-century book), but hopefully it will make more sense when we add in the next pieces of information. It turns out that a series of churchmen, who were witnesses to the events around 540, indulged in the use of biblical metaphor. That is, instead of describing events in clear text, as we might do, they used biblical quotations to convey their message.

ZACHARIAH

Zachariah of Mythilene, whose 12-volume history, compiled in the sixth century, originally covered the 460s to 560s, is complete only to the end of volume nine which ends in AD 536.[16] Of significance for this argument, Zachariah's key volume 10 is missing and much of the rest is fragmentary. However, in one of the fragmentary texts which dates to 556, Zachariah says that what people, and the generation before them, have just been through 'is like the Curse of Moses in Deuteronomy'. Someone referring back a generation from 556 is spanning the period around 540. So what Zachariah is doing is describing the happenings in terms of an existing text from the Old Testament. The key items in Moses' curse are, that you shall be cursed in the city and in the field and in your store.

> Cursed shall be the fruit of thy body and the fruit of thy land ....The Lord shall make the pestilence cleave onto thee ....The Lord shall smite thee with a consumption and with a fever, and with an inflammation, and with an extreme burning, and with the sword (or drought), and with blasting, and with mildew ....The Lord shall make the rain of your land powder and dust: from heaven shall it come down upon thee ....The Lord will smite you with the botch of Egypt, and with the emerods, and with the scab, and with the itch, whereof thou canst not be healed. The Lord shall smite you with madness, and blindness, and astonishment of heart: And you shall grope at noon-days as the blind gropeth in darkness.[17]

It would seem that Zachariah is being quite accurate in his choice of metaphor, this is pretty much what we reckoned must have happened around AD 540. However, Zachariah includes another element as follows:

> ... and the whole land thereof is brimstone, and salt, and burning, that it is not sown, nor beareth, nor any grass groweth therein, like the overthrow of Sodom and Gomorrah, Admah and Zeboim, which the Lord overthrew in his anger and in his wrath.[18]

By using the Curse of Moses to describe the happenings around 540, Zachariah is indirectly incorporating 'brimstone and fire from the Lord out of heaven'.[19] So, Zachariah's choice of metaphor – with fire and brimstone, darkness at midday, famine and pestilence – seems to confirm the 540 bombardment scenario.

GILDAS

Gildas, by long tradition, was not only writing around 540, he is widely believed to have been the only British writer of the mid-sixth century. Because of this unique status, most attention is devoted to his outline of early British history. However, he also uses extensive passages from the Bible to illustrate what may happen to contemporary sinners, effectively making a collage of quotations all of an apocalyptic nature. Here is an example of one of his statements:

> Behold, the day of the Lord shall come…to make a wilderness of the land…the brilliant stars in the sky shall cease to spread their light, and the sun shall be shadowed at its rising ….The moon will grow red, the sun will be confounded ….[20]

Gildas, writing around 540, seems to be drawing together references which relate to a dust veil that affects the light of the sun, moon and stars which in turn produce a 'wilderness.' In recent years, David Everett, who had made a study of apocalyptic literature, went through Gildas' apocalyptic choices in detail. He pointed out a pattern wherein Gildas uses these Old Testament quotations but makes them contemporary, i.e. directly relevant to the period just around 540. For example, here is Gildas making a 'telling aside':

> After a while he [Isaiah] discusses the day of judgment and the unspeakable fear of sinners: 'Howl! The day of the Lord is near' [*and if it was near then, what are we to suppose today?*] 'for destruction is on the way from the Lord' (Gildas' comment; Everett's Italics).[21]

The comment in brackets is one of several where Gildas relates his quotations to contemporary happenings that would be recognisable to his readers. Again, here is Everett making such a point:

> Gildas continues ad nauseam to hammer home his apocalyptic message, and it could only have carried conviction if his contemporaries had had some sort of apocalyptic experience.

And again:

Gildas refers to the immoral actions of Constantine as 'poisoned showers of rain' (28:4), a curious phrase to use unless the population had recently experienced such a downpour. He (also) urges Aurelius Caninus to shake himself 'free of your stinking dusts' (30:3).

THE *IRISH ANNALS*

Once it was realized that this use of metaphor was in vogue around the middle of the sixth century, an attempt was made to find some other examples. Surprisingly there was one in the *Irish Annals* that stood out because of its date. It says:

> The Age of Christ, 539. The decapitation of Abacuc at the fair of Tailltin, through the miracles of God and Ciaran; that is, a false oath he took upon the hand of Ciaran, so that a gangrene took him in his neck [i.e. St Ciaran put his hand upon his neck], so that it cut off his head.[22]

The important point here is that Abacuc is not an Irish name. However, here is someone called Abacuc being killed at Lugh's Fair at Tailltin (Teltown) in 539; Lugh, who we have seen above described as a comet, traditionally founded the fair at Teltown. Who, then, is Abacuc? The answer is that he is Habakkuk of the Old Testament. Hence, what the 'compiler' of the *Annals* was doing, by saying that Abacuc lost his head in 539, is directing his reader to Chapter 3 of the Book of Habakkuk (it is in Chapter 3 that Habakkuk mentions 'Thou smotest down the head in the house of the ungodly, and discovered the foundations, even onto the neck of him.'). In this case, again, we have an anonymous monk using Old Testament metaphor to describe what was going on around 540. So what does Habakkuk Chapter 3 tell us? It includes:

> Before him went the pestilence and burning coals: he ... drove asunder the nations; and the everlasting mountains were scattered .... The sun and moon stood still in their habitation ... the fields shall yield no meat ... and there shall be no herd in the stalls.[23]

Again this seems like a consistent description of what was going on around 540, with pestilence and burning coals from the sky and famine on the ground. In this case, the writer also provides the strong secondary link to Lugh's Fair – the Festival of the comet god Lugh. It could be asked why Zachariah, Gildas and our anonymous Irish compiler do not describe the happenings overtly? There could be various reasons for this, from the conspiratorial 'they were instructed not to do so', to the simple fact that medieval writers did not write like modern journalists. Their scholarship was rooted in biblical tradition; it may have been quite logical to let the available texts speak for themselves. After all, their contemporary read-ers, mostly churchmen, would likely have known these quotations by heart.

If we look back over these various statements, there is a distinct pattern. The references used include the following: pestilence; consumption; burning coals; burning diseases; mildew; powder; dust; botch; scab; itch; brimstone; salt; fire from heaven; dim sun, moon and stars; poisoned showers; stinking dusts and darkness. These are all closely linked to the period around 540 when we *know* we have a dry fog, or dust veil, involved in a global tree-ring downturn, with famines and the outbreak of a severe plague. It looks as if the choices of metaphor are extremely accurate. But, perhaps most interesting are the references to dust (stinking and otherwise), powder and poisoned showers. The reason for this is that Keys was able to locate Chinese references to falls of dust in 535, 536 and 537.[24] While Gibbon provides the strange reference:

> Such was the universal corruption of the air, that the pestilence which burst forth in the fifteenth year of Justinian (AD 542) was not checked or alleviated by any difference of the seasons … but it was not until the end of a calamitous period of fifty-two years that mankind recovered their health, or the air resumed its pure and salubrious quality.[25]

Taken all together, these scattered pieces of information raise the spectre that the air around the globe was corrupted with dust (or some stinking poisoned shower) in the time window 536-45, in the immediate vicinity of 540. Gibbon could not have known that the time period he chose to specify corresponds very closely to the 'Maya Hiatus' of c.AD 534-93.[26] Is that just another coincidence? Overall it looks as if the myths and metaphors get closer to supporting the 'we had a brush with a comet or its debris around 540' scenario than any conventional historical sources.

STORIES FROM OPPOSITE ENDS OF THE OLD WORLD

Having gone through the fact of the 536-45 tree-ring event, and related some of the other material which exists in the literature but which is usually ignored (be it references to comets, corruption of the atmosphere, myth or apocalyptic metaphor) it is possible to imagine the reader saying 'but if any of this were true, surely it would have been recorded by the Chinese who were great astronomers?' This question has been asked numerous times following lectures that touch on this subject. The issue is how to defuse this sort of logical, and apparently damag-ing, question. After all, if these comets and global events were not recorded by the Chinese, it would probably be fatal for the comet scenario in most people's eyes. However, it is known that things were relatively stressed in China just at this time. For example, Margaret Houston referring to the period straddling 536 says:

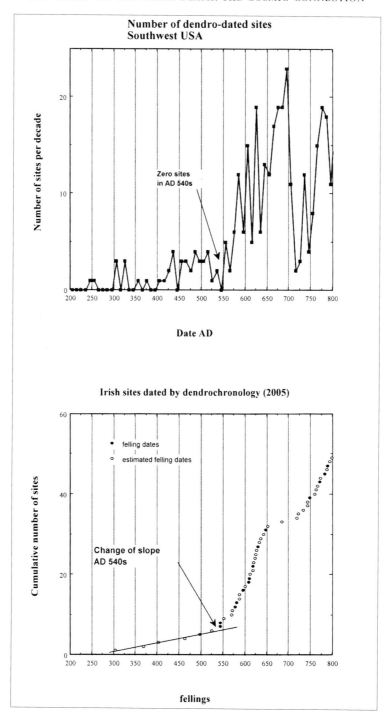

23 Plotting the number of tree-ring dated archaeological sites shows clearly how the 540 environmental event marks a change point in both Europe[27] (below) and the American south-west[28]

Drought combined with other portents led people to question the legitimacy of the three competing Chinese dynasties and in a practical sense it made the government, especially in the north, difficult to maintain. Ethnic origins, political circumspection of resources, and decentralized government appear to have contributed to tensions that precipitated the disintegration of the Wei Empire. The AD 536 event could have contributed to the disintegration of that government and the popularity of other-worldly religions, especially Buddhism.[29]

All in all, with empires disintegrating, perhaps we should not expect good astronomical records to survive in China around 540. Obviously that sounds like a weak argument; clutching at straws to preserve the comet hypothesis. However, this is where serendipity takes a hand. In 2005 Robert Juhl provided a translation of a medieval Japanese document, the *Enoshime Engi* (History of Enoshima Temple).[30] In short, in 1047 a Japanese monk wrote a history of the Temple and, in particular, some happenings just prior to the arrival of Buddhism in Japan. Now, the traditional date for the arrival of Buddhism in Japan is 538 (though Juhl uses 552). Either way, somewhere in the immediate vicinity of 540, there was an apparition of the bright goddess Benzaiten. She was seen to look 'like an autumn moon enveloped in mist'. She was adorned with a long jade pendant and her descent was accompanied by a strumming or slapping sound (given as *Sakusaku taru*). She was accompanied by a myriad spirits of dragons, fire, thunder and lightning that made 'great boulders descend from above the clouds'. In addition, she arrived after an episode 'when dark clouds covered the sky and the earth quaked continuously for 11 days'.

Amazingly, in Ireland, there is the story of *Mongan's Frenzy* which is dated to 538.[31] In this 'fairy' story a bright, long-haired, Celtic god, Mongan, experiences the 'sky going black' before 'a terrible shower of hail stones' drives him, and his colleagues, to seek shelter in the otherworld. This is clearly the same event being described at opposite ends of the Old World. Indeed, if things were falling from the sky as far apart as Ireland and Japan we can only imagine the global scale of the associated disaster – the 540 event! Maybe Roger of Wendover was right after all, when he claimed that a vast comet was seen from Gaul around 540 that made the whole sky seem to be on fire. Indeed he may have been nearly right when he claimed that something – that could be mistaken for real blood – fell from the sky just before a dreadful mortality.

CONCLUSION

If, in the sixth century, metaphors and myths tell us what happened at the time of a global environmental event, when history plainly does not, who are we to believe? And if strange stories (in the sense of myth, metaphor, unsubstantiated and disregarded 'histories') are more accurate than (what passes for) 'history' in the sixth century, who is to say that such stories may not be at least as accurate in the fourteenth century? Here is another hint of the strangeness of the sixth-century event.

It is possible to read Procopius and come away with the impression that the plague started somewhere in Africa in 540 and arrived into Constantinople in 542. Until recently this was a *comfortable* dating because it was also 'known', from the *Irish Annals*, that the 'plague' arrived into Ireland in either 544 or 545.[32] So, in the conventional wisdom, plague broke out around 540 in Africa, was in Constantinople in 542, and had probably arrived in peripheral Europe around 545. This made its spread look very like the conventional wisdom regarding the spread of the Black Death. Hence the bubonic paradigm was preserved; probably the same disease, probably the same rate of spread, probably the same kill rate. However, recently, in a re-analysis of the *Annals*, McCarthy and Breen have shown that this reference to the arrival of Blefed in Ireland is more likely to relate specifically to the year 540.[33] This re-dating would, of course, pull the rug from under the bubonic plague paradigm. If plague arrived into Ireland in the same year that it broke out in Africa then bubonic plague simply would not do. This would raise the spectre of some airborne agent. Something that might sit comfortably with Gibbon's 'corrupted atmosphere' or Wendover's 'bloody rain'. It would sit comfortably with the metaphors of Zachariah, Gildas and our Irish monk, who corporately suggest all the elements from pestilence to stinking dusts, and darkness, listed above. It might even sit comfortably with the proposed loading of the atmosphere with debris from a comet.

So, the only way to get a clear picture of the happenings around 540 seems to be to take account of both myths *and* metaphors. If this was the case for the sixth-century plague, why should not we expect at least a hint of something similar in the weird reports from the time of the Black Death? We have already seen that there are unusual environmental happenings in tree-ring and radiocarbon records in the fourteenth century. We probably need to take more serious note of some of Hecker's 'compendium of Cosmical Upheaval'. In case this all seems too fanciful it is worth looking at the hard evidence deduced from the tree-ring dates for archaeological sites in both Ireland and the American south-west. *Figure 23* shows the results from these two completely independent areas.

EARTHQUAKES
AND OTHER ISSUES

The reader may be surprised by this chapter. It was written at a comparatively early stage in the development of the book. Later a much better handle developed on some of the events mentioned but, instead of re-writing the chapter, it seemed more sensible to leave it largely as it is. That way the reader gets to see how the lines of reasoning developed. The thought process was this. If, as noted in the last chapter, back in the sixth century it is the myth and marginal literature that gives the *best* indication of what may have been going on, then, when we come to consider the fourteenth century, we possibly should not dismiss the weird stuff. We also have to remember that, given the information in the early chapters, our target time window for consideration of what may have caused the Black Death is no longer necessarily restricted to the 1340s. There seem to have been a series of odd environmental goings on, almost from the start of the fourteenth century.

Just what sort of things do we need to consider? Well, there was 'the great earthquake that was felt throughout England on 14 November AD 1318'.[1] While an earthquake might just be a tectonic plate movement, we are forced to remember that England does not often experience severe earthquakes. When they do occur, they are seldom felt 'throughout England' but more usually locally. When there is a widespread earthquake, we have to recognise that, whether we like it or not, earthquakes *do not have to be tectonic*. Yes, they are usually tectonic, but they can be caused by other phenomena. For example, an earthquake could conceivably be due to a distant impact event. We know that very widespread earthquakes would accompany any major impact and it is widely hypothesized that at the extinction of the dinosaurs there would have been a massive 'ground wave' associated with the impact. Obviously we are not looking at any extinction-level event in recent millennia, but even the 1908 Tunguska airburst – with its estimated 15-megaton blast – did shake the ground over a wide area. Tunguska is interesting for many reasons, not least the controversy as to what it was. Most discussion relates to whether it was an asteroid (a solid stony or metallic object) or a fragment of comet.

One very good reason for assuming it was a 40m lump of comet relates to its trajectory, and to the date of its arrival. Both of these parameters are suggestive of it being part of the Taurid complex of comet debris. Here is a little more on Tunguska in case the reader is not familiar with the event.

> The Tunguska meteorite fell at 7.17 a.m. on June 30 1908 .... Its fall was accompanied by exceptionally violent optical, acoustical and mechanical phenomena and even by seismic and aerial shockwaves .... The fall of the meteorite was seen in a cloudless sky over a huge territory of Central Siberia ... i.e. over an area about 1500km in diameter ... there were deafening detonations, which were heard at distances of more than 1000km from the place of fall. Afterwards thunder, crackling and rumbling were heard. Over a huge area...ground tremors were felt, buildings shook, window panes broke, various objects and household utensils fell down, hanging objects were set swinging ...[2]

The event was recorded as an earthquake by seismographs at Irkutsk, some 890km from the blast site, while the aerial shock wave was registered very widely including on micro barograms in six different meteorological stations in England. The fall of the Tunguska meteorite was accompanied by other interesting phenomena.

> The first night after the fall ... was unusually bright everywhere in European Russia and in Western Siberia, as well as in the rest of Europe. Even in the South, for example in the Caucasus, one could read newspapers without artificial light at midnight. At the same time, so-called luminous (silvery) clouds were seen in many places against the background of bright twilight. Subsequent nights were also very bright .... It appears that beginning about the middle of July and extending to the second half of August 1908, an appreciable lowering in the coefficient of the transparency of the atmosphere was observed.[3]

What is most sobering about this set of descriptions is the realization that this is almost *the only known earthquake caused by an impact from space*. It occurred in 1908. People have been producing written records for about 5000 years. It is probably fair to say that every other recorded 'earthquake' in the whole of history is assumed to be tectonic! Could that really be the case? That no other earthquake in history was caused by an impact? After all, we know of several crater fields formed by impacts in the last few millennia. So objects have struck the earth. But, since the exact dates of these impacts are not known (examples would be: the Sirente crater field in Italy which is dated by radiocarbon to around 1650+/-40 before present; this translates to a calendar date somewhere between AD 300-500;[4] the south German crater field formed around 2000 years ago;[5] the Kaali crater field in Estonia dating somewhere between 1500 and 400 BC[6]), it is impossible to say if the earthquakes associated with these impacts were recorded or not.

When this *lack of impact-induced earthquakes* was first thought about, it was realized that it was not just historians that might have a false impression of the level of hazard from space. When scientists read about an earthquake in ancient sources they do not normally jump to the possibility of some of the events actually being impacts from space. Yet if even a tiny percentage of the recorded earthquakes were impact-induced, it would completely change the current (lack of) impact paradigm. Here we need to know about the current state of research on impacts. I'll simplify the story but preserve the main elements because the reader needs to know the nature of the debate that goes on in astronomical circles. The debate boils down to the issue of asteroids and comets. Asteroids are solid bodies of rock and stone, and it is known that about 1000 such solid bodies with diameters of 1km, or more, cross the orbit of the earth. These are Apollo or 'earth crossing' asteroids. There is an American school of astronomers who believe that these bodies are the main threat to the inhabitants of earth. They have made the case that these Apollo asteroids should be found (by photographic survey) and their orbits should be worked out. If all 1000 could be found by survey (and identified as posing no short-term threat) then these astronomers believe that we would be relatively safe for the foreseeable future. Their current reckoning is that the likelihood of being hit by an object this size is about once in 100,000 years.

The reader will see how neat a picture this asteroid threat makes. The astronomers have already found and tracked about 700 of the proposed 1000 Apollo asteroids. None, so far, are likely to hit us in the foreseeable future, and the survey is scheduled to have found 90 per cent of the total population by 2008. However, this would still leave the larger number of bodies which are sized between 100m and 1km. These would need to be found, but these are believed to pose less risk (they would probably not produce a global catastrophe if one were to hit us, whereas something 1km or greater in diameter probably would). This school of astronomers feels that it would be possible, over time (and with improved technology), to survey everything down to a few hundred metres in diameter. If the reader was not previously aware of this issue, it is worth thinking about. Basically what these astronomers are saying is that there are objects that cross the path of the earth but they hardly ever hit us and, moreover, they (the astronomers) are going to make sure we are safe (by safe they mean that if a body is found that in the future might be a threat, they will have time to devise means of defusing the threat by diverting the asteroid away from the earth). In 'asteroid astronomer' world there have not been any serious impacts in the last few thousand years and they are going to ensure it stays that way.

The only problem is that there is another school of astronomers! This school could be called the 'comet hazard' school and it is British based. So what do they think? Well, they think very differently from the American asteroid school. Comets are different from asteroids in that they are made of water ice, frozen gas, organic (carbon-based compounds) materials, and probably odd bits of rock and metal (*Appendix 2*).

As comets pass through the inner solar system they are heated by the sun and outgas thus we see them as bright objects with gaseous tails. If they pass through enough times they can outgas completely and then all that is left is a very black lump (they can be any size and are typically a few kilometres in diameter). The reason they are so black seems to be due to the poly-aromatic-hydrocarbons that are concentrated onto the comet's surface as a tarry coating. These objects are hard to spot because they do not reflect sunlight (in contrast, the asteroids do tend to reflect sunlight which is why astronomers can spot them). In reality the whole business of comets is slightly more complicated than this.

In addition to dying, and ending up as black lumps, some comets leave trails of dust and debris in the inner solar system that the earth passes through. The meteor showers that are seen on various nights of the year are in fact particles from comet trails burning up in the atmosphere. The problem is that comet nuclei can also break up and this gives rise to a hierarchy of potential hazards. Imagine that in addition to any trail of comet dust (such dust would in itself be no problem because any of its particles striking the earth would burn up in the atmosphere) there are large pieces of dead comet scattered along the trail. What happens if one (or several) of these hit the earth? Remember, because they are black no one will see the piece(s) coming. If such hazards exist, they are very hard to do anything about. If we cannot see them how are we supposed to divert them? Worse still, if they do hit us, they will tend not to leave craters; so ancient examples of such impacts will be hard to identify. This means that comet fragments represent a particularly intractable problem for the inhabitants of earth. The dilemma is that one group of these British comet-astronomers believes that there are good grounds for thinking that there are quite a lot of large, dead, comet nuclei orbiting in the inner solar system. Moreover, their concern is that these objects are so black that they are virtually impossible to detect.[7] Compared with the asteroid threat, nothing much is being done about the threat posed by fragments of comets.

Now, let's move to the important point. These comet astronomers believe that the Tunguska object of June 1908 was a fragment of Comet Encke. They would also point to the *fact* of the 20 or so fragments of Comet Shoemaker-Levy 9 that ploughed into Jupiter in July 1994. Where they differ from the asteroid astronomers is that they think such impacts by fragments of comets are quite frequent. They would argue about whether the earth might suffer a Tunguska-class impact once every century, or once every 300 years. They would not, under any circumstances, believe that the earth is safe on timescales of tens or hundreds of thousands of years!

To make this as clear as possible: there are two very, very different perspectives on hazards from space. In one – the asteroid school – there have been very few impacts in the last few millennia. In the other – the comet school – there may well have been numerous impacts by comet debris that have affected human populations in recent millennia. With this background the reader can hopefully now see why issues such as 'how do you tell an impact from an earthquake?' are important. We need to know whether the American asteroid school is right … or if it is wrong, because, *if it is wrong the earth is a much more hazardous place than is currently believed*.

Historians and archaeologists, of course, have not thought about the issue – most probably do not even know the debate exists. It is probably fair to say that researchers in these disciplines exist in an intellectual bubble where there simply are no impacts from space. Environmental researchers – like the current author – are trying to understand global environmental downturns that might have been caused by loading of the earth's atmosphere by comet debris, in a world where historians, archaeologists and asteroid astronomers either do not know, or do not believe, that such things can happen. The problem these three groups face is that the global downturns (as indicated by tree-rings) sit comfortably within the hazard parameters understood by the comet astronomers. Recently, astronomers at Cardiff have noted how a fragment of comet impacting the earth's atmosphere would eject a plume back out into space. This plume would then spread to deposit a debris cloud on top of the atmosphere (this was observed when the Shoemaker-Levy 9 fragments impacted Jupiter's atmosphere in 1994). They went on to calculate how big the fragment would have to be to induce the environmental effects observed in AD 536. Surprisingly, they found that a fragment about half a kilometre in diameter would be sufficiently large to account for the environmental observations.[8]

It seems that when it comes to understanding the impact hazard, the only way to disentangle such phenomena, in historical sources, would be to find some other recorded symptom, or symptoms, that might prompt us to look in the right direction. We shall come back to this whole issue of impacts and earthquakes later.

DISENTANGLING IMPACT PHENOMENA

What else have we got that might help us disentangle some of these past phenomena and separate out the causes of earthquakes? One immediate area for speculation is whether an extraterrestrial impact on, or over, an ocean might trigger both an ocean effect and an earthquake? If there was an impact over the Atlantic we might expect evidence for some tsunami activity to be recorded at the same time, say in England or the Netherlands. The problem is that in the past tsunamis were not described as such. They tended to be described as 'floods' or 'coastal inundations' and were normally assumed to be simple storm surges, or tidalwaves. Worse still, when someone tries to pull together a record of inundations affecting England in the first half of the fourteenth century, as Mark Bailey (that is Mark Bailey the historian *not* Mark Bailey the comet astronomer) has done, lo and behold there is an inundation in roughly half of all years between 1300 and 1350.[9]

Nothing stands out in the flood record to argue for any significant inundation event coincident with our 1318 English earthquake. So, there are no immediate grounds for proposing the possibility of an impact around 1318. However, it is worth considering 1331 because, in that year, we have a record of a whale stranding in Dublin Bay.[10] The good thing about the stranding of whales is that there is a bizarre tradition in China which goes along the lines of 'when comets appear whales die',[11] i.e. sometimes when comets were seen in the heavens, the oceans really were hit by debris and whales were killed (presumably). The other good thing is that a big stranding does suggest that something had acted to interfere with the whales – the stranding acting as a physical manifestation of something going on. Is there an inundation recorded for 1331? Well, yes there is. In 1331/32 there was a severe inundation of the south coast of England associated with both flooding in the Netherlands and, by implication, in Norfolk.[12] One wonders about what went on in 1331, but that is almost all one can do, wonder. Though just to show how much information is out there, an article turned up in *National Geographic* concerning the excavation of a fourteenth-century Chinese sea-going junk. Divers recovered some 200,000 coins and 12,000 artefacts from the wreck which was found off the west coast of South Korea. Here is what they say about the dating:

> The most recent coins found aboard, minted in about 1310, prove that the ship could not have sunk before then. A lacquer-ware bowl bearing four Chinese characters – possibly designating the year 1331 – indicates that it may have foundered very close to that date.[13]

How intriguing to find beached whales and a sunken junk recorded around the same time, and around a time when radiocarbon work hints that the oceans may have been affected by something. Of course, it could be just a meaningless coincidence, but we have no grounds for dismissing the coincidence out of hand. There has to be some possibility that the inundation, the whales and the sinking, were all due to some common cause, and we can envisage a real mechanism that could produce all these symptoms, namely the arrival of a shower of material from space striking the world's oceans.

Hopefully it is clear what is happening. By playing around with the idea that some earthquakes or inundations or freak occurrences, may be signs of impacts from space, one is attempting to move away from the conventional wisdom. If, in an open-minded survey, someone found a record of a fireball on one day, someone else found a record of an earthquake on the same day, while a third person noted an inundation at the same time, then there would be good grounds for linking the pieces up. In reality this proves difficult because of the poor dating of most records. As it happens, no one seems to have recorded anything else on 14 November 1318. But let's keep going.

We could turn to Ziegler who researched sufficiently to write his widely read book on the Black Death.[14] Although Zeigler tends to be dismissive of the 'odd' things that occurred before the arrival of the plague (the 'signs' if you like) he does list a series of them. The following is a paraphrase of the types of phenomena he found:

> droughts, floods, earthquakes, locusts, subterranean thunder, unheard of tempests, lightning, sheets of fire, hail stones of marvellous size, fire from heaven, stinking smoke, corrupted atmosphere, a vast rain of fire, masses of smoke. He discounts reports of 'a black comet seen before the arrival of the epidemic' but still records the warnings: heavy mists and clouds, falling stars, blasts of hot wind, a column of fire, a ball of fire, a violent earth tremor, in Italy a crescendo of calamity, involving earthquakes, shortly before the plague arrived.

It is interesting that there are several references in this list to earthquakes and, indeed, to things 'falling from the sky'. The normal assumption is that these are hysterical ramblings or Old Testament apocalyptic, but there has to be the possibility that there actually were exceptional hail stones, and rains of 'fire from heaven'; it is entirely possible that the sky was a lot more active at some periods in the past. Furthermore, the idea of a black comet is an interesting one. There are several ways in which a comet could appear as 'black', including if it was close enough for the nucleus to be visible to the naked eye. The reason that might be of interest is because it would allow the possibility of the comet passing close to the earth and loading the atmosphere, something that would then link to the 'corrupted atmosphere' idea. Overall, nothing in Ziegler's list is in any way impossible.

It seems that in the 1340s there is a rash of earthquakes. Rosemary Horrox compiled many of the original documents relevant to the period, and her book is a mine of information in this vein. She gives us a writer in Padua who tells us that, not only was there was a 'great earthquake' on 25 January 1348, but it was at the twenty-third hour. He tells us that it was aimed (by God) at terrifying the Christians. This is elaborated as follows:

> In the thirty-first year of Emperor Lewis, around the feast of the Conversion of St Paul [25 January] there was an earthquake throughout Carinthia and Carniola which was so severe that everyone feared for their lives. There were repeated shocks, and on one night the earth shook 20 times. Sixteen cities were destroyed and their inhabitants killed …. Thirty-six mountain fortresses and their inhabitants were destroyed and it was calculated that more than 40,000 men were swallowed up or overwhelmed.[15]

The problem with this particular document is that there are parts one would like to believe and others that seem to stretch credulity. For example, the author goes on to mention a town, Cencenighe, where no one was left alive. If true, that would be interesting because there are few earthquakes where *everyone* is killed. But remember this is a document of dubious credibility. The author mentions that he got some information from 'a letter of the house of Friesach to the provincial prior of Germany'. It is the 'information' in that letter which causes most people to switch off. He says:

> It says in the same letter that in this year [*presumably 1348, if we take it at face value*] fire falling from heaven consumed the land of the Turks for 16 days; that for a few days it rained toads and snakes, by which many men were killed; that a pestilence has gathered strength in many parts of the world .... (This author's italics.)[16]

How does anyone handle such statements? If there was 'fire falling from heaven' at this time, it would be incredibly important information. But, the mention of toads and snakes would occasion most scholars to simply disregard the whole statement. As we've seen, Ziegler repeats this information, but it is pretty clear from his tone that he does not believe it. Let's take a recent writer who has cast a critical eye over the whole plague issue. Samuel Cohn devotes a couple of pages to the issues around earthquakes, toads and snakes. It is interesting to see his tone. He lists a series of very weird happenings, for example:

> ... a dragon at Jerusalem like that of Saint George that devoured all that crossed its path ... a city of 40,000 ... totally demolished by the fall from heaven of a great quantity of worms, big as a fist with eight legs, which killed all by their stench and poisonous vapours.[17]

Then he goes on to repeat a story by the Dominican friar Bartolomeo, who told how:

> ... massive rains of worms and serpents in parts of China (*Catajo*), which devoured large numbers of people. Also in those parts fire rained from Heaven in the form of snow, which burnt mountains, the land, and men. And from this fire arose a pestilential smoke that killed all who smelt it within twelve hours, as well as those who only saw the poison of that pestilential smoke.[18]

Now consider his tone. After reporting the above he says:

> Nor were such stories merely the introductory grist of naïve merchants and possibly crazed friars ...[even]... Petrarch's closest friend, Louis Sanctus (Socrates), before embarking on his careful reporting of the plague ... claimed that in September floods of frogs and serpents throughout India had presaged the coming to Europe in January of the three pestilential Genoese galleys ...[even]... the English chronicler

Henry Knighton …[reported how]… at Naples the whole city was destroyed by earthquake and tempest. Numerous chroniclers reported earthquakes around the world, which prefigured the unprecedented plague. Most narrowed the event to Vespers, 25 January 1348.[19]

Clearly he is surprised that even respectable people are reporting this stuff. He might have expected it from some 'crazed provincial friar', but Socrates, for heaven's sake, that is hard to believe. Then his tone changes; he reports the next list 'dead pan':

Of these earthquakes that 'destroyed many cities, towns, churches, monasteries, towers, along with their people and beasts of burden, the worst hit was Villach in southern Austria (Kärnten)'. Chroniclers in Italy, Germany, Austria, Slavonia, and Poland said it was totally submerged by the quake with one in 10 surviving.[20]

Obviously earthquakes are acceptable in a way that 'fire from heaven' is not. After all, many different chroniclers refer to this earthquake event, so it has a comfortable reality to it. So how does he deal with the (above) problem of respectable people saying crazy things about dragons and poisonous worms and fire from heaven? Well, he gets out of it cleverly. First, he points out that all this stuff was being reported purely as 'manifestations of God's ire'. This was because people in the late 1340s obviously saw the issue in such terms. But, fortunately, and this is Cohn's tone, it was as if a little later the chroniclers all 'got better'; they 'wised up'. He points out how historians often use this 'crazy' information to provide a picture of the 'plague's fantastic and religious origins', but:

What they fail to report is just how fast this 'aetiology' [meaning 'search for cause'] of plague faded with successive strikes ….After 1350, we hear no more of the floods of snakes and toads, black snows that melted mountains, or the presage of earthquakes, and little of astrology or even God.[21]

How does one put this: 'and with a single bound, he (Cohn) was free?' It is a masterly treatment. Cohn has managed to *mention* the craziness (because, of course, he, and everyone else, has to), but, in reality, it was just that at the start of the plague people did not understand anything and, as they desperately flailed around looking for *causes*, they just reported all this weird stuff. Then, when they started to get a handle on the issue of treatment, and realized it was just a severe disease (not sent by God at all), by about 1350, they caught themselves on, and thereafter wrote normally. Thus, having dealt with the issue Cohn moves on to later plagues and more comfortable ground. Do not be mistaken, Cohn's is a remarkable book. However, on this issue, as far as can be seen, he takes the same tone as Ziegler, and just about everyone else. People wrote about earthquakes, 'fire from heaven' and 'floods of toads and snakes' but we *know* it was just hysteria. Put another way, if you want to keep working as an historian, you had better believe it was just hysteria! Again, we shall return to these issues later.

IMPACTS AND TSUNAMI

It seems that we might need to be more open-minded when interpreting historical information. When is an 'earthquake' actually a symptom of an impact and not just a tectonic event? When is a 'coastal inundation' actually an impact-induced tsunami and not just a storm surge? If, as the comet-astronomers suggest, the earth is hit by comet debris much more often than asteroid-astronomers believe, how do we test the suggestion? The answer is that we have to be aware of the very wide range of information that might be necessary to disentangle the evidence. We also have to recognise that there is a real issue out there. Impacts from space by comet debris could have played a significant role in the history of the last few millennia. The written evidence may have to be read in a new and more open-minded way if we are ever going to make sense of it. At this point it is perhaps worth commenting further on the recently discovered south German crater field at Chiemgau. A scientific literature is now developing on the subject. It is claimed that the impact was in the Celtic period, i.e. 2000-2500 years ago, and that the incoming object was a fragment of a comet.[22] The evidence is impressive, and indicates that there is nothing fanciful about the idea of impacts by comet fragments in recent millennia. We are left with the question of exactly when the Chiemgau event occurred; and the secondary question as to whether or not an earthquake was recorded at the same time. As another example of the type of information that is out there, take the case of Australian tsunami. Ted Bryant has studied some of the bizarre coastal formations around the coast of Australia. Bryant is an academic coastal geo-morphologist. He has stated things that seem so farfetched that his statements are usually ignored. For example:

> Perhaps the most dramatic deposits are those containing piles of imbricated boulders. These piles take many forms ....At Jervis Bay, New South Wales, blocks weighing almost 100 tonnes have clearly been moved in suspension (i.e. lifted by high velocity tsunami waves) and deposited in this fashion above the limits of storm waves on top of cliffs 33m above present sea level.[23]

The idea of 100 tonne boulders being hoisted and set down on the tops of 33m cliffs by tsunami is well outside normal human experience. But, in point of fact there is no good reason for ignoring the physical evidence. The problem is that tectonically induced tsunami just will not do as an explanation for the placement of such boulders. Observed *tectonic* mega-tsunami, such as the one that affected

Indonesia and Sri Lanka on Boxing Day 2004, have singularly *failed* to emplace
huge boulders on 30m-high cliffs. Faced with this, Bryant has had to consider
what it *would* require. The answer in his view is that it would require a significant
impact over an ocean to provide the necessary high-velocity waves. Bryant has
dated numerous tsunami deposits around Australia (*24*) and finds:

> Six separate tsunami events can be recognised over the last 8000 years, with peaks at
> 7500 BC, 5000 BC, 3300 BC 500-2000 BC, AD 500, and at AD 1500 ....The peak of the
> AD 1500 tsunami event corresponds with the largest number of meteorite observa-
> tions for the past two millennia. In addition, the peak at AD 500 corresponds with a
> clustering of meteor sightings that is believed by astronomers to be one of the most
> significant over this time-span .... Both of these clusterings are associated with the
> Taurid complex.[24]

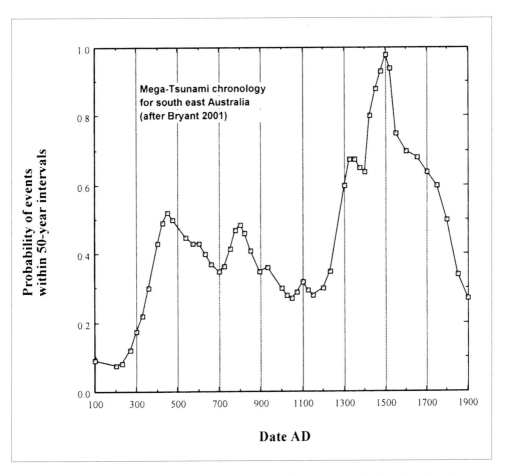

24 Ted Bryant's plot of the probability of tsunami based on a range of radiocarbon dates for
tsunami deposits around Australia

It does not take a genius to see what is being said here. The bizarre Australian tsunami deposits cannot be tectonic in origin; they must have been produced by impacts over the oceans. Some of the clusters of tsunami dates then coincide with peaks of meteor sightings; and we know meteors are streams of comet debris. QED embedded in the streams of comet debris are objects (like the Tunguska object, or even bigger) big enough to cause the tsunami that deposit the huge boulders on the high cliffs. Currently most academics lack the necessary multi-disciplinary approach (or the open-mindedness) required to appreciate such information. It is perhaps easier to ignore it and hope it goes away. However, the lesson of Boxing Day 2004 is that the Indonesian tsunami, big and all as it was, *cannot have been even remotely* the biggest tsunami in recent millennia. Bryant has evidence for tsunami that were definitely bigger, they occurred in recent mil-lennia, and they were almost certainly produced by impacts not earthquakes. It is probably not coincidence that two of the environmental events discussed in Chapters 5 and 6 fall at 3200 BC and AD 540, while the chosen period of this book relates to AD 1350; dates close to three of his tsunami peaks.

CONCLUSION

Hopefully, at least some readers who have previously soldiered through Chapters 5 and 6 will recognise in this chapter shades of Roger of Wendover. Roger had heard or read of 'a close comet at 540, with a rain of blood, followed by a dreadful mortality'. He was not believed. He was called a fantasist, but it would appear that he was about as right as it is possible to be. It is pretty clear that we should not be ignoring the seemingly weird writings from around 540 or 1348. Indeed, we shall see in Chapter 17 that even those references to showers of toads and snakes should not be dismissed out of hand. Nor should we be ignoring the seemingly unpalatable evidence produced by researchers like Ted Bryant. Recently he has received support from researchers in Spain/Portugal who point out that 'In the last 7000 years, at least twenty tsunami have been registered in southern Iberia'.[25] Like impacts, tsunami events are probably under-represented in any non-cata-strophist view of the world. But ultimately all such factors will have to be fitted into the *real* history of this planet. Without it we are relegated to viewing kings, priests and warriors acting out their little dramas on some *benign* planet that never actually existed.

MORE ON EARTHQUAKES

Let's play around with some of the issues introduced in Chapter 7. Let us imagine, for the sake of argument, that there was a core of truth in the hysteria associated with the arrival of plague in the years 1348 and 1349. If that was the case, then people observed things falling from the sky, including fire. They observed earthquakes, and a general corruption of the atmosphere. They observed a pestilence which was remarkable for its virulence in that its kill rate was unlike anything they had previously experienced. Jon Arrizabalaga, who studied educated writers relating to this same, initial, 1348-9 period, states the following:

> Most of the physicians whose works have been studied here conceived of the *pestilentia* as a universal air condition and attributed it to celestial causes.[1]

Ziegler puts it like this:

> This concept of a corrupted atmosphere, visible in the form of mist or smoke, drifting across the world and overwhelming all whom it encountered, was one of the main assumptions on which the physicians of the Middle Ages based their efforts to check the plague. For one chronicler the substance of the cloud was more steam than smoke. Its origin was to be found in a war which had taken place between the sea and the sun in the Indian Ocean. The waters of the ocean were drawn up as a vapour so corrupted by the multitude of dead and rotting fish that the sun was unable to consume it .... So it drifted away, an evil noxious mist, contaminating all it touched.[2]

So, expert historians, with in-depth knowledge of this period, consistently rehearse this information thereby confirming its existence. There is undoubtedly a corpus of material suggesting that the air was corrupted, due to some celestial cause, with a strong hint that the ocean was involved. This seems like a good point to add in parts of the report of the Medical Faculty of Paris, prepared on the orders of the French king. The report, according to Horrox, was produced in October 1348, and it refers quite pointedly to corruption of the atmosphere associated with earthquakes. Here is part of what they said:

> Another possible cause of corruption, which needs to be borne in mind, is the escape of the rottenness trapped in the centre of the earth as a result of earthquakes – something that has indeed recently occurred.[3]

It seems that the French medics were aware of a recent *series* of earthquakes. Presumably this series included the 25 January quake. But, there is a lot more of interest about this report. Here is an extended quote:

> However, in the judgment of astrologers plagues are likely, though not inevitable, because so many exhalations and inflammations have been observed, such as a comet and shooting stars. Also the sky has looked yellow and the air reddish because of the burnt vapours. There has also been much lightning and flashes and frequent thunder, and winds of such violence and strength that they have carried dust storms from the south. These things, and in particular the powerful earthquakes, have left a trail of corruption. There have been masses of dead fish, animals and other things along the sea shore and in many places trees covered in dust … and all these things seem to have come from the great corruption of the air and earth.[4]

This sounds like pretty authoritative stuff. However, Ziegler thinks that while their report is undoubtedly the most prestigious, it is 'neither the best informed nor the most intelligent'.[5] That statement fits well with the general dismissal of all the 'strange' information from 1348 and 1349. We have already seen two separate statements: one, relating to the Indian Ocean and one to (presumably) the Atlantic coast; both referring to masses of dead fish and corruption. Remember that in the last chapter it was suggested that earthquakes might possibly be the result of impacts from space, rather than tectonic movements. Here we have French medics, writing at the time, mentioning a comet and shooting stars, flashes, violent winds and earthquakes. Each of these elements would be entirely compatible with Tunguska-class impacts. If such an event took place over an ocean we could expect dead fish (and other things) so that fits as well. If a distant eyewitness saw a comet or asteroid entering the atmosphere over the Indian Ocean, it would appear as bright as the sun (as was the Tunguska fireball and explosion). Would a description invoking 'a war between the sun and the sea' be a *bad description* of such an event? Would the description just possibly class as a *metaphor*? Is another possible reason why chroniclers stopped referring to all this 'strange' stuff after 1350 simply that all the comets, meteors, wars involving the sun, earthquakes and corruption had stopped or reduced in quantity? Perhaps, during 1348 and 1349, all these things had been taking place, just as described by a wide swathe of chroniclers. It seems like a perfectly reasonable supposition.

DATING

The second point about the report of the Paris Medical Faculty is in something they say about the plague itself:

> We have not said that the future pestilence will be exceptionally dangerous, for we do not wish to give the impression that it will be as dangerous here as in southern and eastern regions.[6]

When doctors in Paris make such a statement it raises a serious question as to where the plague was in October 1348. It reads as if the plague had not reached Paris when they were writing. Yet Horrox tells us that it had reached Paris by June 1348[7], and Cohn says:

> Finally, according to testamentary gifts to the parish of Saint-Germain-l'Auxerrois in Paris the Black Death rose abruptly in August and probably peaked either in September or October.[8]

So when did the plague reach Paris? Was it June, August or October? There is a difference. You would think that when a pestilence noted for its unusual severity has arrived, it would be pretty clear just when that was. Why is there so much confusion? To confound the situation, Horrox gives us a strange, and interesting, description. According to the *Chronicle of William de Nangis*, in August 1348:

> … a very large and bright star was seen in the west over Paris, after vespers, when the sun was still shining but beginning to set. It was not as high in the heavens as the rest of the stars; on the contrary, it seemed rather near. And as the sun set and night approached the star seemed to stay in one place, as I and many of my brethren observed. Once night had fallen, as we watched and greatly marvelled, the great star sent out many separate beams of light, and after shooting out rays eastward over Paris it vanished totally: there one minute, gone the next …. But it seems possible that it presaged the incredible pestilence that soon followed in Paris.[9]

Again it does not sound as if plague had arrived in Paris by August, just as it seems not to have arrived by October 1348. Interestingly, Twigg also says that 'Klebs asserts that it broke out in Paris soon after October 1348'.[10] It seems inconceivable that people would not have known whether a plague, noted for its virulence, was, or was not, present. But here we have the city of Paris with doubt over

June, August, October or even 'after October'. That has to be bizarre and we shall return to this issue of dating below.

Going back to the content of the 'bright star' record, the writer, who claims twice in the text to have been an eyewitness, makes it plain that some time elapsed while this object was in view; possibly several hours. He even hazards a suggestion that the object might have been a comet or some sort of condensed vapour. What are we to make of it? Might it have been ball lightning or even some low angle bolide, or a peculiar nova? Who knows? But any way it is viewed it adds a 'strange star' to the list of comet, meteors, flashes, falls of fire and a 'sun like object' which clutter 1348.

Let's now take a look at the chronology of the spread of plague across 1348 and 1349, and, as, a starting point, let's take it that there is no doubt about the date of the earthquake of 25 January 1348. Here we have a fixed date to work from. Now let's mine Horrox' compilation for relevant dates. The earthquake predates the arrival of plague in England by a mere five months if we accept that it arrived in Bristol around 25 June 1348.[11] However, there is another date for its arrival in Bristol, namely 1 August 1348.[12] If we accept the story of its arrival at Melcombe, Dorset, then it was 7 July 1348. It may seem like splitting hairs but to a chronologist there is quite a difference between 25 June and 1 August. Late June is the time of the intersection of the earth's orbit with the Taurid meteor stream (remember Tunguska was 30 June), whereas the first of August is the festival of Lugnasa; the festival of the Celtic god Lugh. So, there is a hint in these dates that we might be seeing a mixture of chronology with astronomy *and* mythology. The point, though minor, is an interesting one.

The real problem is that none of these dates need be correct. This is because as late as 17 August 1348 the Bishop of Bath and Wells is instructing his archdeacons to pray that the pestilence which 'has arrived in a neighbouring kingdom [presumably France]' will be turned away and that 'healthy air' will be sent.[13] This is an excellent example of what we are up against. Some sources have the plague in south-west England by late June, or early August, 1348. Yet here we have an important cleric, in a precisely dated document, seemingly contradicting the idea. It is quite revealing to see exactly what he says:

> Almighty God uses thunder, lightning and the other blows … to scourge the sons he wishes to redeem. Accordingly, since a catastrophic pestilence from the East has arrived in a neighbouring kingdom, it is … to be feared … a similar pestilence will stretch its poisonous branches into this realm.[14]

Surely there is no way to read this text and believe that plague had arrived in England by 17 August 1348. How could the Bishop know about plague being in a neighbouring kingdom and not know that it was just a few tens of miles away? In fact, come to think of it, how was the message transmitted to the Bishop that plague was in the neighbouring kingdom? Presumably some traveller must have taken the risk of introducing the disease to England in order to bring the message? Does this imply that, despite the threat of plague, people were still travelling freely around Europe in mid-1348? If we put this problem together with the Paris problem we are inevitably left wondering about the chronology of the spread of this plague. If the plague was not in Paris in August 1348, and was not even going to be in the city by October 1348, where would this leave all those nice contour maps that are trotted out to illustrate the spread of the plague? Seriously compromised it would seem. Just before pushing this chronology issue a little further, look again at the Bishop's statement. Why does he use the quite specific 'thunder, lightning and other blows' form of words for God's scourge? In fact is there anything in this prayer to suggest that he is talking about disease at all? Later, in his instructions he encourages abasing and prayers:

> … so that the mercies of God may speedily prevent us and that he will, for his kindness sake, turn away from his people this pestilence and the other harsh blows … and send healthy air.[15]

There are those 'harsh blows' again and a tangential reference to corrupted air. What blows is he referring to? Why was he referring to the need for healthy air? Had the information from France, that informed him that pestilence was spreading there, also contained the suggestion that it was corrupted air that was responsible? Or, was the unhealthy air already in England before the plague arrived? (We shall see later that if we take Hecker literally, this also seems to have been the case in Cyprus.) Reading these various contemporary documents it seems quite reasonable to raise the question 'was the pestilence actually poisoned air and not a disease vector at all? The sheer flexibility of the chronology of these early documents allows this sort of speculation. We shall see later what a more plausible solution might be.

Does all of this mean that plague had not arrived into either France or England by mid-August 1348? Could we start to conjecture that the plague in both France and England actually arrived *after* a series of earthquakes; and *after* a strange star performed in some way over the Atlantic? We could reasonably ask if there were any inundations in August 1348. As always, there are plenty of questions, but few answers.

PUSHING THE DATING ENVELOPE

In some ways this would be a good place to stop trying to make sense of the chronology of happenings during the first wave of the Black Death. Any attempt is let down by the failure of chroniclers to systematically record the exact days and times of events. However, there is a need to add in a few more points about the suggested arrival dates of the plague in different areas, in order to raise additional questions. It is probably significant in itself that no clear picture can be deduced. Casting around for somewhere to start, it seems to be generally accepted that the mortality was widespread in the eastern Mediterranean in 1347, and entered Italy and France possibly early in 1348. What follows is the result of a trawl through the compilations by Horrox and Cohn to show how bad things are when we try to understand what was happening in northern Europe (it is not possible for an outsider to go back to the original documentation; luckily these historians have already done this for us).

We have already seen the contradictions about when plague arrived in both Paris and England. When we turn to London, things are very similar. It seems that plague was still not in London by 24 Oct 1348,[16] but it is asserted that it had arrived there by about All Saints (1 November) 1348. On the other hand Cohn tells us that it was either in London by 29 September or possibly one month later at All Saints.[17] Either way it was bad by February 1349 and on through to 12 April 1349. It then, according to one source, *stopped* in London at Pentecost (31 May) 1349.[18] (How do you get a plague to stop? Did the last infected flea in London – if there were any infected fleas in London at all – finally die on 31 May? See *Appendix 3*.) However, again, another source says it ran on until 1 August 1349.[19] It then went north from London, stopping in the north at Michaelmas (29 Sept) 1349. What makes this even more strange is that again, apparently, in Austria the plague lasted from Pentecost (31 May) 1349 to Michaelmas (29 Sept) 1349.[20] If that is correct, we have something peculiar happening that is seldom remarked upon. People have been very interested in when the plague *started* in various places, they seem to have been a lot less interested in when it stopped. Here we have suggestions that it started in Austria just when it stopped in London, and stopped in Austria at the same time it stopped in northern England.

Hopefully the reader can see why playing around with dates is both intriguing and frustrating. They do not seem to make a lot of sense. But here is what may well be the best bit. There is a continental text that dates to Sunday 27 April 1348, which includes the following statement:

> They say that in the three months from 25 January [1348] to the present day [presumably 27 April 1348, when the text is dated], a total of 62,000 bodies were buried in Avignon.[21]

Let us imagine that this precise date 25 January 1348 did indeed mark the arrival of plague in Avignon. If that was the case, then we would have it arriving at the same time as (apparently on the same day as!) the 25 January 1348 earthquake. Now, that is interesting! It is interesting, not least, because this date occurs again

in a German treatise which Horrox thinks was probably composed in the generation after the 1348-9 plague outbreaks. This treatise says:

> Insofar as the mortality arose from natural causes its immediate cause was a cor-
> rupt and poisonous earthy exhalation, which infected the air in various parts of the
> world .... I say it was the vapour and corrupted air which has been vented – or so to
> speak purged – in the earthquake that occurred on St Paul's day, 1347 [*Given that in
> the fourteenth century dates in January were normally referred to as the previous year, the year
> ending not on 31 December but on March 25, we can assume this is actually the earthquake
> of 25 January, in the calendar year 1348*], along with the corrupted air vented in other
> earthquakes and eruptions, which has infected the air above the earth and killed
> people in various parts of the world. (This author's italics.)[22]

So, someone at the time noted this January 1348 coincidence of earthquake and
infected air. How might an earthquake cause 'infected air' in any immediate fashion? At first sight it is hard to see how this could be. However, if we were to
imagine that the earthquake was merely a symptom of, say, an impact (rather than
the earthquake being the prime mover), then we could have the infected air being
introduced coincident with the earthquake. While this may sound far-fetched, it
would fall reasonably well within that (normally disregarded) suggestion by Hoyle
and Wickramasinghe that the plague bacillus *P. pestis* may have drifted down from
space. One does not have to believe their whole thesis, merely take the significant
point they make about the oft-presented contour map of the spread of plague
(credited to E. Carpentier). They suggest that the contours of this spread map do
not make a lot of sense with respect to the movement of an insect-spread disease.
In fact they put it more strongly. They say that the suggested contours 'are a clear
indication that *P. pestis* hit Europe from the air'.[23] So, the simple act of speculating
that the 1348 earthquake might be a *symptom* rather than a cause, leads one to ask
a question that then resonates, just a little, with the considered thoughts of Hoyle
and Wickramasinghe; a pair not to be taken lightly.

Curiously there is another piece of information which just might be significant
in this consideration of impacts possibly being recognised only as earthquakes.
Ziegler mentions the arrival of the plague in the Aegean islands and Cyprus, and
notes that in the second year, which must be 1348, it was killing large animals
such as dogs and horses and all manner of birds, as well as humans and rats. His
source, the Greek historian Nicephoros Gregoras, should have been a reliable
witness because he had seen the plague at first hand in Constantinople in 1347.
Ziegler continues with this comment about the plague:

> While the plague was just beginning a particularly severe earthquake came to com-
> plete the work of destruction. A tidal wave swept over large parts of the island,
> entirely destroying the fishing fleets and olive groves .... A pestiferous wind spread

so poisonous an odour that many, being overpowered by it, fell down suddenly and expired in dreadful agonies. 'This phenomenon,' exclaimed the German historian Hecker in justified surprise, 'is one of the rarest that has ever been observed.'[24]

Now, that has to be doubly interesting. Clearly from both Hecker's tone and Ziegler's endorsement this was a very unusual event. But we know that earthquakes are quite common. We also know that earthquakes cause tsunami and thus tsunami cannot be all that uncommon. Presumably *the thing that is uncommon* is the 'pestiferous wind' spreading a poisonous odour that kills in dreadful agonies. The curious thing is that an impact from space could cause (i) an earthquake; (ii) a tsunami; (iii) a strong wind; and (iv) a poisonous odour. The latter factor is a reasonable possibility given the known presence in comets of poly-aromatic-hydrocarbons (*Appendix 2*).

Now, of course, the problem as always is chronology. If we knew the day of the earthquake in Cyprus it might be possible to make a story (especially if it happened to be 25 January 1348). As it is, it appears to merely represent a curious fact; something to file away. Except, that is, for one thing. Ziegler's extract from Hecker does not capture the *correct* tone. Here is an extract from Hecker:

> On the island of Cyprus, the plague from the East had already broken out; when an earthquake shook the foundations of the island, and was accompanied by so frightful a hurricane, that the inhabitants … fled in dismay …. The sea overflowed …. Before the earthquake, a pestiferous wind spread so poisonous an odour, that many … expired in dreadful agonies … and as at that time natural occurrences were transformed into miracles, it was reported, that *a fiery meteor, which descended on the earth far in the East, had destroyed everything within a circumference of more than a hundred leagues, infecting the air far and wide.* (This author's italics.)[25]

Frankly that is a quite different tone! If this version of Hecker is accurate, then the earthquake did not take place 'just as the plague was beginning', rather 'the plague had already broken out' before the earthquake. In addition, strangely, the poisonous wind was also *before* the earthquake. But, the wind is separate from the 'frightful hurricane' that *accompanied* the earthquake. This seems to be a totally different picture from the one painted by Ziegler. Moreover there is the mention of a '*fiery meteor*' which destroyed, at face value, 24,000km^2 of somewhere to the East. This sounds remarkably like a Tunguska-type blast which destroyed 10 times the area of Tunguska itself. We should probably take note of this 'fiery meteor' that Hecker just happens to drop into the general time-frame of the Cyprus 'earthquake'. It is outright speculation but what if that fiery meteor was actually on 25 January 1348? If that were the case, then the impact would have coincided with an earthquake that was felt all the way from Cyprus to Avignon.

Going back to the issue of dates, let's now go back to Ireland. Horrox tells us of the plague, that:

> It first began near Dublin, at Howth, and at Drogheda [both on the east coast] …. In Dublin alone 14,000 people died between the beginning of August and Christmas [1348] …. In Avignon in Province … it began in the previous January [1348].[26]

That all sounds very straightforward, except, of course, these dates would make it possible that plague arrived in Ireland before it got to either Paris or London. Turning to Cohn:

> In Ireland, according to the sermon diary of Richard FitzRalph, Archbishop of Armagh, plague reached Drogheda about August 1348 and peaked in autumn …. The Franciscan John Clyn reported the same arrival date for Dublin and said it continued to Christmas. For his own village of Kilkenny, however, the mortalities mounted later in the winter of 1349. The chronicler who continued John's work also noted 1349 and not 1348 as the year of the plague's first Irish strike.[27]

Let's see what we can rescue from this mess of confused dates. The one repeated assertion is that plague was present in Ireland by August 1348. But we've already seen that it is questionable whether plague was in either Paris or London, or, indeed, England (remember the Bishop of Bath and Wells) by August 1348. We could add that, from a separate line of enquiry, plague was certainly in Bordeaux by August 1348.[28] That piece of information at least makes sense. Ireland was probably in contact with Bordeaux as part of the wine trade so if plague was in Bordeaux in August 1348 it would seem reasonable that it would get to Ireland around the same time. However, if that were the case, one would have expected plague to have got to London around the same time; yet London was not affected until either late September or late October 1348. All of this raises some interesting questions about the nature of transmission. Why was the whole western seaboard not affected in a systematic way? Why did the north of England need to be infected from London rather than from any number of western coastal ports? As noted previously, what was the vehicle by which the Bishop of Bath and Wells was informed of plague in the 'neighbouring kingdom'?

On reflection, it seems that the most important piece of all this northern European information is the confirmation it appears to give to the date for the arrival of plague in January 1348 in Avignon. This is because January in Avignon gives that link to the 25 January earthquake. It does seem that after that earthquake everyone did go a bit crazy for the duration of 1348 and 1349. Record keeping turned into a shambles, and, as Cohn says, people were blaming God and talking about meteors, earthquakes and corrupted atmosphere, before they 'got better'.

A DIFFERENT SLANT

We have already seen how Jon Arrizabalaga has taken a detailed look at the earliest university-educated writers about the Black Death. He looked at several sources, such as Jacme D'Agramont (Lerida 24 April 1348); Gentile da Foligno (Perugia before 18 June 1348); and Giovanni della Penna (Naples 1348). So his work is an attempt to understand what educated people were writing about the Black Death in its first throes, i.e. before they had any understanding of what it was. His article contains the following discussion on one of the terms used in 1348 by medical practitioners in the Latin Mediterranean.

> One ... Jacme d'Agramont, discussed it in terms of an 'epidemic or pestilence and mortalities of people' ('epidímia ho pestilència e mortaldats de gents') which threatened Lerida from 'some parts and regions neighbouring to us' .... Agramont said nothing concerning the term *epidímia*, but he extensively developed what he meant by *pestilència*. He gave this latter term a very peculiar etymology, in accordance with a form of knowledge established by Isidore of Seville (570-636) in his *Etymologiae*, which came to be widely accepted throughout Europe during the Middle Ages. He split the term *pestilència* up into three syllables, each having a particular meaning: *pes* (= *tempesta*: 'storm', 'tempest'), *te* (= *temps*: 'time'), and *lència* (= *clardat*: 'brightness', 'light'); hence, he concluded, the *pestilència* was 'the time of tempest caused by light from the stars.[29]

Now that has to be pretty amazing. We have been contemplating, albeit speculatively, the plague having something to do with loading of the atmosphere from space. Here is someone (apparently the earliest university-educated writer to look at the plague) writing in April 1348 (well before the plague got to places like Paris or London) using the term *pestilència* in the sense of 'the time of tempest caused by light from the stars'.[30] What is going on? Hecker says that a fiery meteor had destroyed everything within a circumference of more than a hundred leagues, infecting the air far and wide, and d'Agramont says that *pestilència* means 'the time of tempest caused by light from the stars'. Both of these statements were made at essentially the same time. Perhaps we are getting somewhere. Note also that the sense in which *pestilència* is used harks back to the time of Isidore of Seville, just after the happenings of the sixth century, where, again, a cosmic connection is sensed around the time of a 'plague' (one wonders if by 'plague at the time of Justinian' did they also mean *pestilència* ... in the sense of 'something coming on us from the stars' [as stated by Cassiodorus in 537], or in the sense of 'the death of Arthur, an aspect of the god Lugh?').

CONCLUSION

It is fair to say that the two years 1348 and 1349 can be classed as something of an enigma for the simple reason that the type of information recorded about those two years is different in character from that of later years. Cohn has helped enormously with his comment relating to 1350 and how, after this date, we no longer hear so much about 'meteors, earthquakes and corruption of the atmosphere'. The logic of this discussion, on the possibility of earthquakes sometimes being symptoms of impacts, is that in 1348 the earth may have been subjected to a much larger Tunguska-type impact (or impacts) that caused a corruption of the atmosphere as well as an earthquake. We have to ask: what are the chances of developing an argument that January 1348 might, because of the earthquake, be an impact event and then finding that a nineteenth-century writer had actually suggested a large impact in that very year? It looks as though we may have the answer already.

9

BACK TO THE TREE RINGS

It should by now be apparent that, for some reason, record keeping in 1348 and 1349 is simply inadequate to allow sensible study of what went on. Historians have been trying to see through this muddle for what can only be described as 'a long time', without much success. We could point again to the way Cohn despairs of 1348 and 1349 with everyone seemingly blaming God and talking about meteors, earthquakes and a corrupted atmosphere. So it seemed sensible to try a different tack, namely go back to see if there is anything further that can be extracted from the tree-ring records. One approach might be to go back to the tree-ring chronologies and use information from them to attempt to define some key dates in the run up to 1348.

It is possible to treat tree-ring data in different ways, some of them very simple in concept. For example, if we take two neighbouring regions, say Ireland and England, and look at chronologies for oak from those two regions we see a reasonably consistent pattern. Most of the time the two chronologies act pretty similarly, good growth in one region seems to parallel good growth in the other, and vice versa (i.e. the tree-ring patterns go up and down together).

However, occasionally these chronologies will show different responses, wide rings in one region will be mirrored by narrow rings in the other. This is quite powerful information, because the trees that make up the chronologies tend to be relatively long lived. Thus they are represented in the chronologies for long runs of time. This suggests that when the chronologies behave in an opposite manner, the driving force is not the trees but the climate acting on the trees. Put very simply, this opposite behaviour between English and Irish oaks suggests that some environmental boundary has shifted; it is as if someone has drawn a line down the middle of the Irish Sea on a weather map. Trees that were broadly doing the same things suddenly behave in an opposite manner.

A good example of this is presented by happenings just around AD 900. This is another excursion away from the fourteenth century, but it serves to illustrate the way in which an earlier event could be illuminated by looking at tree responses. We can then apply the same idea to the fourteenth century. It had been observed that from the 870s to the 910s English and Irish oaks did behave in a remarkably *different* fashion.[1] The English chronology had been built by Ian Tyers and Cathy Groves. *Figure 25* shows the effect. When this was first observed, it was assumed that it represented some sort of 'end effect' because there had been problems building a chronology in Ireland across AD 850.[2] However, examination of the individual ring patterns across the 870-910 period indicated that the chronologies were adequately replicated and the trees showed no unusual behaviour. Thus the implication was that the differences illustrated in the figure were genuine responses to a change in climate zones. We could also see that, by comparing the

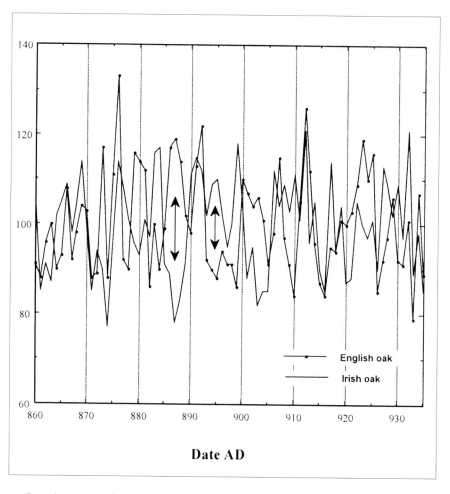

25 Opposite response between Irish and English oak chronologies in the later ninth century; some noticeable offsets indicated by arrows. *English data courtesy of Ian Tyers and Cathy Groves*

two chronologies with others from Europe, it was the Irish trees that were behaving 'differently'. The English chronology continued to agree well with assorted European oak chronologies.

Once sensitized to the fact the something environmental was going on across the 870s to the 910s, it was interesting to observe the following. Bjorn Gunnarson and his colleagues had built a long pine chronology in Central Sweden. The trees used were mostly recovered from lakes. Now, this sounds a bit unusual because trees do not grow in lakes. What seems to have happened is that these trees had grown beside lakes and, after death, some had fallen into the lakes and been preserved. In total, by sampling trees from many lakes, the dendrochronologists managed to build a continuous chronology from 1633 BC to the present. Continuous that is, except for one gap between 887 and 907.[3]

Knowing this, it was a bit of a revelation to see that in a new temperature record, produced by studying the proportion of the oxygen-18 isotope in Greenland ice, there was a notable cold event just across 880-920.[4] Now, when it gets notably colder in Greenland we could reasonably expect that something might be going on in the North Atlantic, or even more widely. *Figure 26* shows how it was easy to find relevant global information. In China the culturally rich Tang dynasty (618-906) ended just around this time. Moreover, the Tang was not succeeded by the stable Sung dynasty until 950; in between is the chaotic, troubled five-dynasty period. In Central America the long-lived Maya civilization was finally ended by a succession of severe droughts. The *very last* Maya inscription dates from around 910.[5] Reference to *Figure 26* shows just how coherent the picture is. It may have been cold in Greenland, but the manifestations of this apparently global upset can be seen in different ways in different areas.

We could reasonably ask what caused this event (or eventful period). Here, as usual, we are left with no obvious cause. If we look at Britton's compilation we find that in this 40-year period there are reported: gales and thunderstorms, inundations, a number of what may have been aurora, and even two 'showers of blood'.[6] The problem, as always, is that none of this information is particularly out of the ordinary. It does not give any clue that might explain the changed conditions recognised by the oaks. The important point is that a period picked out by the opposite growth response of oaks turns out to be part of a bigger picture.

APPLYING THE SAME IDEA TO THE FOURTEENTH CENTURY

If we plot the same Irish and English oak chronologies across the fourteenth century (27) we see that from 1300-6 the trends in the two chronologies are very similar, e.g. both chronologies picking up the reduced growth in 1303 and 1304; in the following years, 1305 and 1306, both chronologies show increasing

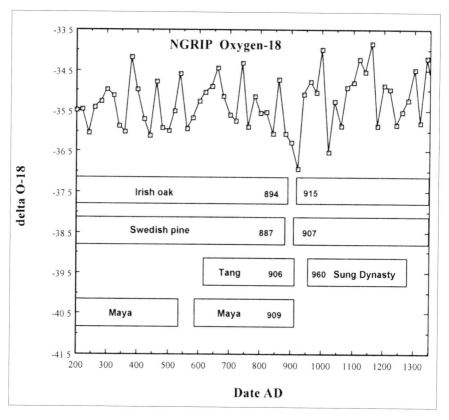

26 Gaps observed during chronology construction in Ireland and Sweden coincident with reduced temperature in Greenland. The collapses in Tang China and the Mayan civilization are also indicated. *Temperature data courtesy of J.P Steffensen*

growth. However, the next four years, 1307-10, show distinctly opposite growth trends. Although this opposite response is not as dramatic as that seen across AD 900; nevertheless, it indicates a change of some sort around 1306-07. At the very least it indicates some type of climatic alteration on the fringes of the Atlantic. As soon as this is noted it jogs the memory that the Dublin medieval oak chronology runs from 855-1306. Not a lot to go on but interesting because many years of sampling failed to extend the Dublin area chronology forward in time beyond 1306. It has never been clear why 1306 marked the latest date of any oak timber on the extensive Dublin medieval excavations, though logic would suggest that *something* must have changed.

In the two chronologies, the 1312-7 mean widths are similar, 1318 and 1319 are opposite. Then from 1320 through to 1353 the trends in the two chronologies are surprisingly similar. This is a reversion to the 'normal' situation where Ireland and England exist in the same climate regime, as far as oak trees are concerned. Looking just at these two regional chronologies we get an impression of disturbance in 1307-

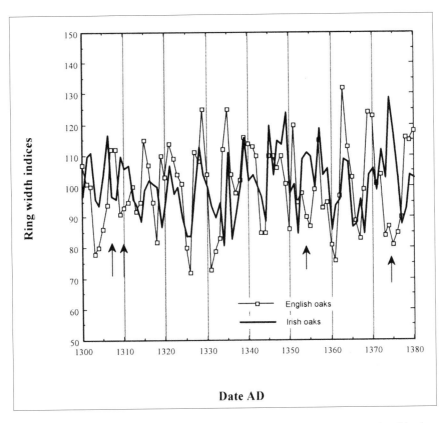

27 Notable opposite responses in Irish and English oak between 1307-12, 1354-6 and in the 1370s; other single year offsets are in 1319 and 1334. *English data courtesy of Ian Tyers and Cathy Groves*

10, and 1318-19, then stability until another pulse of opposite behaviour in 1354-56. So, this 50-year period contains three notable departures from normal. To put this in context, after 1356 there is only one notable divergence between the Irish and English chronologies (at 1374-7) in the whole period 1356-1620. This is a different way of looking at historical quality events, and it does give us a feel for this new type of information. Clearly agreement is the normal situation; these opposite departures represent abnormal conditions of some description.

To pad out this picture we can go back to some information from Chapter 2. There we saw that in the 1320s and 1330s we had a sudden cooling of the North Atlantic surface water, simultaneous with an abrupt downturn in European oak growth. When we look again at the plot of sea-surface temperature (*28*) it is apparent that there is a radical change in character of the chart after 1320. It is noticeable that the sea-surface temperature from 1300 to about 1318 oscillates on a high frequency – two to three year – cycle. Suddenly, after 1318, the record enters 15 years, from 1319-33, where it goes from this rapidly changing mode to

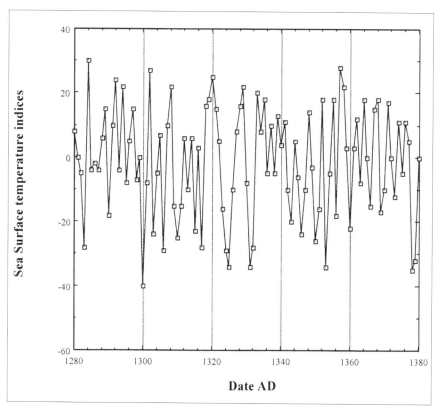

28 The reconstructed North Atlantic sea surface temperature showing altered character in the 1320s and 30s. *Data courtesy of Alastair Dawson*

one that is smoother and longer-term. The character is clear in *Figure 28*. After 1333 the rapidly changing mode returns.

So, now we have:

Oak opposite behaviour Ire/Eng 1307-10; 1318-9; 1334; 1354-6; 1374-7
Longer cycles in sea-surface temperature 1319-33; 1356-60; 1377-80

Given that the opposite behaviour is deduced from tree-ring patterns, while the cycles are derived mostly from the Greenland ice, it is interesting that the years 1319, 1333-4, 1356 and 1377 represent 'change points' in both records. Obviously, as this book is aimed at issues relating to the half-century running up to the Black Death, the change-point dates that are most interesting are 1307, 1310, 1318-9 and 1333-4. To that we can add the pairs of cold years 1324-5 and 1331-2. If we open up Ziegler's book on the Black Death, or indeed one of any number of others on the topic, we find that they consistently rehearse the main facts from Hecker's nineteenth-century work on the subject. Hecker had stated that:

... simultaneously with a drought and renewed floods in China, in 1336, many uncommon atmospheric phenomena, and in the winter, frequent thunderstorms, were observed in the north of France; and so early as the eventful year of 1333 an eruption of Etna took place. According to the Chinese annals, about 4,000,000 of people perished by famine in the neighbourhood of Kiang in 1337; and deluges, swarms of locusts, and an earthquake which lasted six days, caused incredible devastation. In the same year, the first swarms of locusts appeared in Franconia, which were succeeded in the following year by myriads of these insects. In 1338 Kingsai was visited by an earthquake of 10 days' duration; at the same time France suffered from a failure in the harvest; and thenceforth, till the year 1342, there was in China a constant succession of inundations, earthquakes, and famines. In the same year great floods occurred in the vicinity of the Rhine and in France, which could not be attributed to rain alone; for, everywhere, even on tops of mountains, springs were seen to burst forth, and dry tracts were laid under water in an inexplicable manner. In the following year, the mountain Hong-tchang, in China, fell in, and caused a destructive deluge; and in Pien-tcheon and Leang-tcheou, after three months' rain, there followed unheard-of inundations, which destroyed seven cities. In Egypt and Syria, violent earthquakes took place; and in China they became, from this time, more and more frequent; for they recurred, in 1344, in Ven-tcheou, where the sea overflowed in consequence; in 1345, in Ki-tcheou, and in both the following years in Canton, with subterraneous thunder. Meanwhile, floods and famine devastated various districts, until 1347, when the fury of the elements subsided in China.[7]

Now, if we put that list in chronological order and add in the additions from Ziegler we have:

1333 eruption Etna

1333 parching drought and famine followed by floods in China

1334 drought followed by locusts, famine and pestilence

1336 drought and renewed floods in China

1336 uncommon atmospheric phenomena and frequent thunderstorms in France

1337 serious famine, deluges, locusts and a six-day earthquake in China

1337-8 locusts in Franconia

1337-45 earthquakes, floods, locusts and 'subterraneous thunder' in China

1338 harvest failure in France

1338 10-day earthquake in China

1338-39 high death rates in Central Asia

1338-42 constant inundations, earthquakes and famines in China

1342 floods in Germany and France (rain and tectonic causes)

1343-7 assorted earthquakes, deluges, inundations and subterraneous thunder

1348 fiery meteor

Writers on the Black Death, from Deaux,[8] through Ziegler to Cohn, and others, all repeat this information, but make no real objective comment upon it. It is as if they either do not believe the information, or they treat it as hyperbole, or they treat it as unsupported, or they have no way to relate it to anything other than the general sentiment that 'environmental issues got rodents on the move, taking the pestilence with them'. Certainly it is hard to find any writers who have attempted to wring any sense out of this list. But, of course, until recently no one has had access to the information given by tree-rings, radiocarbon measurements, and ice cores. We can look at this list with a fresh eye.

For example, it has to be *of interest* that the lists of calamities mostly start in 1333. We can now see that this is not an arbitrary date, because of the flip in bristlecone pine growth, in America, after two decades of good growth, to a period of more than three decades of relatively poor growth (*20*). The mid-1330s is also our best estimate for the change in the radiocarbon calibration curve from ^{14}C enrichment to depletion (Chapter 3). It seems to be replicated in a change of mode in the North Atlantic sea-surface temperatures. We could reasonably ask what happened in or immediately after 1333. It would also seem reasonable to suggest that the climate upsets in China (1333 parching drought and famine followed by floods) are reflected in changed conditions on the other side of the Pacific, as well as in the North Atlantic region. So, it does look as if there is a global component to whatever was going on. However, just because the upset may have been global does not mean that everywhere was *badly* affected. For example, in 1333 crop prices in England actually fell dramatically.

CONCLUSION

Changes in tree-ring responses can be used to highlight climate differences between regions. The observations around 900 served to illustrate the point. It is then possible to use the same idea to draw out some changes in the fourteenth century. Some of the dates for 'change' are then found in other records, to the extent that a picture can be built up across time. It is clear that something profound happened around 1333. This was already known from the radiocarbon calibration work (Chapter 3) and from the bristlecone pine chronologies and the work at Arroyo Hondo (Chapter 4). The disturbed nature of the period from 1330 to the late 1340s was already indicated by evidence from the south-eastern river-flow reconstructions (Chapter 4) and this can be added to as follows:

In 1342 there were very serious floods affecting the whole of Germany.[9]
In 1345 Tasmanian huon pines indicate the third coldest year in three millennia.[10]
In 1345 Siberian larch indicates the sixth coldest year in several millennia.[11]

So, objective records indicate a major environmental change around 1333 with the following two decades being characterised by disturbance. It is just in this same period that the Anasazi ran into problems in the American south-west.

This same episode, 1333-47, was highlighted many years ago by Hecker as a calamitous period. His information is often repeated, but seldom thought to be of any real significance. Yet we now know that his assertions are backed up by this new science-based information. So, why should we not believe most of what Hecker said? On balance he seems to have found the correct tone in his descriptions and it now seems reasonable to suppose that there is a core of truth in the pre-1348 information that he supplied. Of critical importance is whether his 'fiery meteor' statement is part of the 'core of truth'.

10

CHANGING GEAR

Study of the past is hamstrung if it assumes that the world is a level playing field, and that what we experience today is what people experienced in the past. Here is an example that illustrates the nature of the problem. Since about 1978 it has been acceptable to discuss the demise of the dinosaurs, around 65 million years ago, in terms of a catastrophe brought about by an impact on the earth of a large comet or asteroid. It became acceptable because in 1978 the Alvarez father and son team published real evidence, in the form of a worldwide iridium anomaly at 65 million years ago, to support the impact hypothesis.[1] However, well before 1978 the possibility of an impact as cause was widely discussed, as were about 100 other hypotheses which included everything from loss of sex drive, to thinning (or thickening) eggshells, to the radiation effects of a nearby supernova etc., etc. Even in the 1970s the impact hypothesis was easily the most attractive – after all we only have to look at the Barringer crater in Arizona to see that hard objects do hit the earth. Thus, when the Alvarez paper came out, it seemed that we knew the answer – 'it was an impact that had wiped out the dinosaurs'. It has been interesting, therefore, to watch the ebb and flow of the debate on dinosaur extinction over the last quarter of a century. The same old arguments, and ideas, are trotted out just as they were in the decade before 1978. This seems to be because people like to play devil's advocate, but also because people in academia have careers to build. They need to publish papers and go to conferences. So re-hashing the old arguments about the dinosaur extinction, and trying to dream up new possibilities, helps to keep a lot of people in career-building mode.

Why mention this on-going debate? The reason is that it illustrates the difference between science and historical study. In science you are allowed to throw ideas at issues and see if they make any sense. The difference between historical and scientific debate is that scientists seem to be willing to look at a wider range of possibilities, even outlandish ones. This is valid because, of course, we know little or nothing about the sorts of things that have happened in the past; all we have is the patchy historical record.

We have to face the fact that back in time the written record is totally inadequate for reconstructing the kinds of thing which might have affected human populations, particularly environmental happenings. So, for example, in the past people had no idea of what was happening *far away*. Our modern world view, where a bus accident in Australia, or a rail crash in India, or a landslide in Chile, is transmitted instantly to everyone on the planet, is totally unlike the situation even in the recent past. In the days of sail, let's say up until the later nineteenth century, news could take weeks to travel. For a lot of the world, even quite major events would go unrecorded.

Many readers may scoff at this last paragraph. 'Of course, we have a good idea of what happened in the past,' they'll say. Such a view may be mistaken. Take this example from the ice-core records. If you access the particulate record from the American GISP2 ice core, you find that they give both the numbers of particles in the ice and the size of the particles through time.[2] They provide this information running back to the seventh century. If you look at this 1300-year record you discover that the section of ice with the *most* particles and the *largest* particles is in 1920-2. This spike is so huge in comparison with anything else in the record that it stands out like a sore thumb. There is a lesser but still outstanding spike at 1916. What on earth was the 'event' that caused this 1920-2 anomaly? One could possibly understand something in the middle of World War I putting dust into Greenland, but it is hard to think of a 'once in 1300 years' happening around 1920. Thus, as recently as the 1920s, when the world was well connected, we have a complete enigma involving anomalous amounts of coarse dust – someone might like to solve this little enigma! Examples like this one (and there are many, many others relating to past happenings) suggest the past really is a bit of a mystery.

Building on that thought, let's try another tack. Take the following hypothetical example. Let us *imagine* that, in the year AD 1014, a 200m object travelling at 30,000 miles per hour impacts the south Atlantic. The resultant 100-megaton explosion would have been a world-class event, probably with environmental consequences. The question is would it have been recorded in the historical record? The answer is at worst, no, and at best, tangentially. This is because of a hierarchy of problems with the recording of distant environmental events. First, there would have been no eyewitnesses to such an explosion; anyone in line of sight of the impact would probably have been fried. Second, there was no intellectual foundation for any understanding of such an event, with the result that even 'over the horizon' observers would have had no clue as to what might have happened – flashes and thunderous noises, earth tremors, even fireballs traversing the sky, would have been no guide. So, in all likelihood, no one within 1000 miles of the impact would have been in a position to record that an object had hit the earth. Further away this disconnection between the actual event and any physical effects would have been even more pointed. All that would have been recorded would have been weaker secondary effects such as peculiar weather conditions, or possibly strangely bright nights.

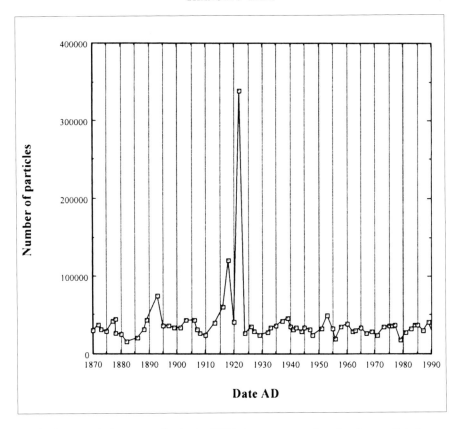

29 The large particulate anomalies in the GISP2 ice core around 1916 and 1921. *Data from: The Greenland Summit Ice Cores CD-ROM. 1997. Available from the National Snow and Ice Data Center, University of Colorado at Boulder, and the World Data Center-A for Paleoclimatology, National Geophysical Data Center, Boulder, Colorado*

However, an impact over an ocean would almost certainly have produced a tsunami. The tsunami could travel enormous distances, so technically it might have been recorded somewhere. Here a major problem comes to the surface. Any distant observer seeing a tsunami coming on shore would have had no reason to identify the marine incursion as an impact-induced tsunami. Given that, at distance, the tsunami might only be a few metres high, it would, at best (because at worst it will not be recorded at all) have been misinterpreted as a 'freak wave' or an 'inundation'.

This is the nature of the problem for, say, historians (indeed for everyone). If all one looks at is the historical record, there may be a complete mismatch between the nature of things that actually happened and the distant descriptions that may be the only surviving written traces – a 100-megaton impact (a global-class event) might be recorded only as a localised coastal inundation 8000 miles away. But, not every coastal inundation is the result of a 100-megaton impact from space, so trying to extract relevant information is essentially impossible.

THE REAL AD 1014 EVENT AND THE REDUCED ACID STORY

Imagine that a scientist has some *independent* reason for looking at the year 1014. Perhaps because there is a suggestion in some scientific data that something strange and environmental may have taken place in that year (in the same way that one is now forced to go looking for an explanation for the 1920-22 particulate anomaly). This is exactly what happened when the ammonium record in the GRIP ice core from Greenland was accessed in *The Greenland Summit Ice Cores CD-ROM* (a data source that is also available on the Web).[3] The reader now knows, from Chapters 5 and 6, that there are good grounds for being interested in anything that happened around AD 540. When the GRIP ammonium record was searched, lo and behold, was not there a distinct ammonium layer at a depth of 336.325m in the record. The ice-core workers have dated this anomaly by counting the annual layers of ice back from the present and arrived at an age of 1410.9 years before 1950; which translates to AD 539.1. Scanning through the record, one has to go back to about 150 BC to find another value as high as this. However, more interestingly, as the record is scanned forward in time, there is only one *higher* value and it occurs at depth 237.875m. This depth translates to AD 1015.4. However, just to add a bit of complication, in this case there is also an elevated ammonium value in the next core section down, at depth 238.425m dating to AD 1012.7. How does one put a date on such an event? Well, as a start, let's take an average of the two estimated dates; that gives 1014.05 (let's call it AD 1014). We are now left with a scientific fact:

> The largest concentration of ammonium in the twenty-two-century time interval between AD 1642 and 596 BC is in the layer of ice centred on AD 1014, in the GRIP core from Greenland.

What on earth causes the largest concentration of ammonium in over two millennia of record? The answer, scientifically, is that no one knows for sure, but some explanation is required. Scientists have cast around for likely vectors and have decided that ammonium in the ice is most probably the result of 'biomass burning', i.e. the result of major forest fires.[4] However, if that were the case one would have to ask what on earth caused the *biggest* forest fire in two millennia? Most of the effort to identify the source of ammonium in the ice-cores has been concentrated in the last century or so. It is clear from the question marks in the titles of the published papers that there is no absolute certainty in this attribution of ammonium to forest fires. Indeed, in one article it is stated that the ice-core workers 'believe' this to be the case.[5]

It has been thought for quite some time that ammonium also occurs in comets. For example, Lyttleton suggested this as early as 1953.[6] Sagan and Druyan were of the same opinion,[7] while Chandra Wickramasinghe stated that the presence of the amino group (NH$_2$) in the emission bands of cometary coma and tails made it reasonable to assume the presence of ammonia.[8] In fact, there is now direct evidence (*Appendix 2*). Large amounts of ammonium were detected in Comet Hale-Bopp by studying radio emissions as the comet passed closest to the sun. It was estimated that, compared with the water content of the comet, ammonium made up around one to two percent (i.e. if there were 100 units of water in the comet, there were one or two units of ammonium; since water is a main constituent this would still imply a lot of ammonium).[9] Is there any mechanism for getting ammonium from a comet into the earth's atmosphere? The answer has to be 'probably'. However, ammonium, for all we know, may be generated by high-energy events in the atmosphere, due to incoming bolides or fireballs, i.e. by the fireball effectively cracking the gasses in the atmosphere. Ammonium is produced commercially from nitrogen and hydrogen subjected to high temperature and pressure, in the presence of a catalyst. It is easy to imagine in the high-pressure, high-temperature, conditions of a bolide impact, that ammonium

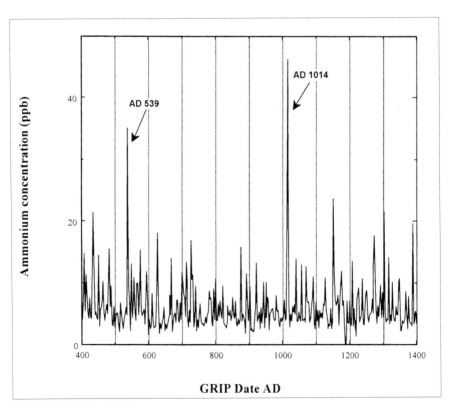

30 The ammonium record in the European GRIP ice core showing the large spikes at AD 539 and 1014. *Data from: The Greenland Summit Ice Cores CD-ROM. 1997. Available from the National Snow and Ice Data Center, University of Colorado at Boulder, and the World Data Center-A for Paleoclimatology, National Geophysical Data Center, Boulder, Colorado*

might be produced directly by incoming objects from space. This last paragraph is a classic example of scientific speculation. The question is whether any of the speculations can be made to stand up; in this case it just so happens that we have something approaching a 'smoking gun'.

This smoking gun takes the form of the Tunguska event of 30 June 1908 (that we looked at in Chapter 7). Although it was frustrating that the European GRIP ice record was not available between AD 1642 and the present, searching through the available data disclosed that there was another record from the American GISP2 ice core. To clarify, while the GRIP core was analysed in 55cm sections, from 1642 back to around 850 BC, the American GISP2 core was analysed at more than one resolution. The available, high-resolution, GISP2 record is discontinuous, but with a little searching it is possible to find that, at a depth of 33.3404–33.4034m, there is an enormous amount of ammonium.[10] This translates to the ammonium occurring somewhere in the middle of 1908. In fact, when we see that the age of the central point of the measurements was at 1908.48, that's as near as one can reasonably imagine to 30 June 1908, just when the Tunguska object entered the atmosphere and exploded. There are also high levels of chlorine, nitrate (nitric acid) and sulphate (sulphuric acid) in exactly the same layers of ice, but from the point of view of this discussion it is the ammonium that is important. The American analysis shows us that, irrespective of the mechanism involved, a high-energy event in the atmosphere seems to have led to a significant amount of ammonium being deposited in the ice record. So, if Tunguska caused an ammonium anomaly in 1908, then, when we go back to 1014 and 539, impact events have to be a *possible* explanation for the large ammonium spikes there. Just to elaborate a little, ammonium was not the only nitrogen-based compound produced by the Tunguska impact. It has been estimated that the high-energy impact event generated 30 million tons of nitric oxide in the atmosphere. In turn, this has been shown to have annihilated about one third of the earth's protective ozone layer.[11] It seems that incoming space debris could well be a source of both ammonium and nitrate in the Greenland ice record.

These pieces of chemical information suggested that the impact idea might just stand up to scrutiny. This, in turn, led to a search for other evidence. In the case of 1014, Britton in his meteorological compilation found two useful facts that seem to be related to this year. First, there was an inundation:

1014 Severe Marine inundations on September 28

Anglo-Saxon Chronicle: And in this year on St Michael's mass eve came the great sea flood widely through this country, and ran so far up as it never before had done, and drowned many vils [*places where people live*], and of mankind a countless number. (This authors italics.)[12]

That has to be interesting, because, as has already been suggested with respect to earthquakes, a major sea incursion – and the *Chronicle* does make it sound pretty exceptional – could be caused by one of a number of possible vectors including an impact from space. Although it does not prove the case, it is encouragingly in the right direction. Let's put it this way. When an ammonium anomaly gives rise to the possibility of an impact, and this dovetails with a natural event that could also be the result of an impact, it is reasonable to give the possibility serious consideration. This is further enhanced when Britton's second entry is considered.

> 1014 Short refers to a remarkable calamity in this year. He says 'a heap of cloud fell and smothered thousands'. He adduces the *Anglo-Saxon Chronicle* as authority for this phenomenon, a work in which there is certainly no mention of it. It might conceivably be a poetic distortion for a heavy rainstorm in which many people were drowned.[13]

Clearly Britton could not make any sense of this strange reference by Short; indeed, his tone is positively dismissive (though it is a bit hard to see how he managed to get from a 'smothering heap of cloud' to a 'rainstorm'; his suggestion can only be described as weak). We now have the independent evidence that this reference to 'a smothering heap of cloud' coincides with an anomalous atmospheric concentration of ammonium. So instead of dismissing the reference as unsupported, we can now, with some reasonable certainty, assume that the report is probably correct. A heap of cloud probably did fall in 1014, and probably did smother thousands of people.

Is there anything else that might improve our understanding of this 1014 event? What makes 1014 particularly intriguing is that the date is listed by astronomers Sekanina and Yeomans as a year when a comet made a relatively close approach of the earth.[14] Once a comet comes close to the earth, the danger of colliding with fragments becomes a real possibility. So, there is a close comet in the general vicinity at the right time; something again broadly supportive of the impact hypothesis. What is almost as important, however, is another story from China. The story would, because of its content, normally be regarded as a myth, and hence it would normally be dismissed out of hand. However, as was shown in Chapter 5, in several other catastrophic events, such as those around 2350 BC, 1150 BC and AD 540 myth can actually be a good guide to what happened. Here is how this Chinese story goes.

THE CHINESE POST–1012 EXTRATERRESTRIAL VISITATION

This story is a little complex but it goes more or less as follows. If you are interested in a date such as 1014 you can pick up a book on Chinese mythology and leaf through to see if that date occurs anywhere. Prior experience with the myths associated with strange characters – immortals, sky deities, gods and spirits – that were around at the time of the Battle of Mu in the twelfth century BC (Chapter 5) helped in this regard. So, leafing through Derek Walters' book *Chinese Mythology* it was no real surprise to spot an *eleventh-century date* associated with a story about the Jade Emperor, Yü Huang.[15] The story says that the Chinese emperor Chen Tsung (AD 998-1023) was accused of having 'invented' Yü Huang (The Lord of Heaven) in order to promote his own authority as a seer. Such a clearly mythic story would normally be skipped over because it sounds irrelevant to anything in the real world; however, because of the ammonium clue that there may have been an extraterrestrial visitation, it seemed worth soldiering on. The main thrust of the story can be followed up in Werner's book on Chinese myth.[16] There it says that in the tenth moon of 1012 (i.e. late 1012) the Chinese emperor Chen Tsung claimed to have had a dream in which he was visited by Yü Huang (The Lord of Heaven) who said he had already sent down two missives, but was now going to follow this up by sending down an ancestral immortal named Chao. It is recorded in the story that 'a little while after, the ancestor came'. Not a bad find; looking for the date 1014 and finding a story of something being sent down from the sky 'after late 1012'.

The thing about these myths/stories is that it is necessary to have some inkling as to how to handle them; this is where previous experience can help enormously. Because of prior interest in the twelfth century BC, there was an awareness of the character No Cha or No Chia who was present at the time of the fall of the Shang (he is mentioned briefly in Chapter 5 under 1159 BC). Basically, Werner tells us that the Chao who descends from the sky 'after late 1012' is the sky deity No Chia, who wreaked havoc back in the twelfth century BC.[17] We have already seen that there is a story linking the twenty-fourth and twelfth centuries BC, and another from the AD 670s referring back to the twenty-fourth-century 'flood' (Chapter 5). Now we have a story linking the twelfth century BC to a date 'after late 1012'. Three catastrophic events linked by myths form a convincing argument that the myths do indeed preserve a core of truth.

We now have the exciting possibility that an ammonium spike in the Greenland ice, around 1014, coincides with the descent of a smothering heap of cloud, and an inundation. This possibility is now backed up with a Chinese story, where a deity of chaos is sent down from heaven around the same time, and just to round the story off, mainstream astronomers testify to the relative proximity of a comet around the same time. So, what answer would the reader like?

(i) An impact from space brought ammonium directly from a comet fragment and also produced a tsunami (noted as an inundation) or,

(ii) An incoming object from space produces ammonium in its high-energy interaction with the atmosphere (rather like Tunguska), and also produced a tsunami (noted as an inundation).

The real problem is that most historians exposed to such deliberations will probably say – 'come back when you have the answer' – i.e. they do not want to indulge in speculation, they want 'proof'. The scientist on the other hand needs help to try and come up with the scenario which might ultimately lead to proof – he or she wants hints as to what the real answer may be, and is, in a sense, appealing to historians to 'read between the lines' in order to come up with hints of what might actually have happened on some occasions in the past. The feeling of the present author is that possibility (ii) makes the most sense given the way this particular story is building up.

SOME TREE–RING INFORMATION POSSIBLY RELEVANT TO THE DATE 1014

Readers will remember the compilation of 1300 tree-ring dated sites (involving 27,000 individual dates) from the American south-west mentioned in Chapter 4.[18] There we saw that the decade of the 1350s showed a reduction in site construction in an area which should not have been affected by plague. A review of the long list of dates quickly ascertained that if we take the 100 years from 915-1014 there are 86 sites represented. If we then take the next 100 years from 1015-114 we find 230 sites. So, somewhere around the early eleventh century there is a significant change in the rate of site construction in the American south-west. *Figure 31* shows the resultant plot. It is pretty clear from this diagram that somewhere in the vicinity of 1014 something changed in this part of America. It does not much matter what the 'something' was. For our purposes it suffices to suggest that, at around the time of a peculiar environmental happening in 1014, with hints from the British Isles to China, something also took place in the Americas. Since the Old and New Worlds were isolated from one another at that time, again the common vector has to be an environmental one.

As always, in this sort of speculative research, one casts around to see if there are other examples that might conform to the fireball/ammonium model. One other date between 539 and 1014 stood out; in the GRIP ice record there is an ammonium layer at AD 626. This date had been pointed out previously by Michael Purser after a lecture in Dublin. He had observed, in frescoes relating to the Siege of Constantinople in 626, that there were 'stars falling from the sky' associated with a disturbed sea that could easily be an attempt by the artist to indicate a tsunami.[19] This is the thing about this developing story; more and more strands of evidence seem to fit comfortably with the idea of impacts from space. Falling stars in a painting mean nothing in themselves. However, when it is a painting of a *dated* event, and the Greenland ice has ammonia at that same date, then the falling stars and disturbed sea possibly take on a whole new significance.

CONCLUSION

Given that there was a pre-existing argument that the events around 540 seemed to involve extraterrestrial impact,[20] we now have strong indications that there are four occasions in the last 1500 years, 539, 626, 1014 and 1908, where we can link dated layers of ammonium in Greenland ice to suggestions of high-energy atmospheric interactions with space debris. Why is all this stuff about impacts being addressed to readers of a book about the environment in the run up to the Black Death? Well, there is some method in the madness. If there is a sensible connection between ammonium and extraterrestrial bombardment, it seems reasonable to ask if there is any evidence for unusual levels of ammonium in

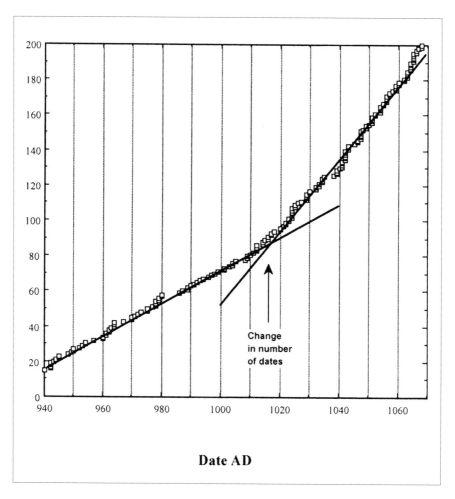

31 Running sum plot of the tree-ring dates for archaeological structures in the American south-west showing the turning point around AD 1014. *Data compiled by William Robinson and Catherine Cameron*

the fourteenth-century ice. We shall come back to this issue in a later chapter. However first we need to expand a few more things that readers need to know in order to make sense of the full story.

THE LEWIS CHAPTER

EARTHQUAKES AND IMPACTS

It is now necessary to make another apparently tangential excursion, and to go back to an issue raised in Chapter 7, namely how some 'earthquakes' in the past might have been produced by impacts rather than tectonics. In the years immediately after the collision of comet Shoemaker-Levy 9 with Jupiter in July 1994 a whole series of astronomical writers produced books on impact hazards. SL9 had acted as a sort of wake-up call to the scientific community about the threat posed to planets, including ours, by asteroids and comets. One of these books in particular, *Rain of Iron and Ice* by John Lewis, was a decidedly scary read. The part of the book which is particularly relevant here is a section which produced a series of impact 'scenarios'. Basically, Lewis looked at what we know about impacts, and said this:

> We know with certainty that stones of all sizes, from centimetres to tens of metres, bombard the earth in modern times. We know that many bodies, like the Tunguska bolide, explode with extreme violence in the atmosphere and leave no lasting geological evidence ….We know from spacecraft missions to the Moon and Mars what the average rate of cratering has been in the inner solar system in recent times … (we have) powerful proof of the bombardment of Venus by comets and asteroids and the selective destruction of smaller and weaker impactors by explosions in the dense atmosphere, giving us a valuable check on our theories of explosions in earth's atmosphere.[1]

Obviously he gives relevant detail. However, from the perspective of this book, the above quotation carries the main message, i.e. that the earth is regularly hit and many of the impacting bodies, like Tunguska, explode in the atmosphere without leaving either craters or any long-lasting visible evidence. But, just because such past impacts have not left craters does not mean that effects on the ground will necessarily have been negligible. Lewis, taking what we know about the range of possible impactors, frequencies, etc., generated what he called 'a statistically reliable computer model' of the typical behaviour of the myriad objects that orbit in our proximity in the inner solar system. Put simply, he produced a computer program that mimicked the likely bombardment of the earth over time. He then ran the computer model many times, looking at 100-year time intervals, in order to assess the level of variation that might 'be expected from one century to the next'. In the book he detailed 10 consecutive one-century computer runs (his scenarios A to J) and, just to concentrate the mind, he told each scenario's 'story' as if the 100-year interval was the twentieth century.

What was startling about these scenarios was that there were four 'centuries' out of the 10 in which the earth was hit multiple times by megaton-class explosions, and yet the fact that they were extraterrestrial in origin went unrecognised! The way Lewis puts it is like this:

> In an average year there is one atmospheric explosion with a yield of 100 kilotons or more. The large majority occur in such remote areas, or so high in the atmosphere, that they are not observed. Even if observed, the witnesses may see only a flash of light in the distance, or hear the 'rumble of distant thunder' coming from the open oceans. Thus even those that are observed are often not recognised.[2]

But, let's not be misled by that quotation. Note that it is only relating to a typical *year*. In his 'century' runs the results included:

> Scenario A: one 10.9-megaton explosion at 3km altitude and 6 megaton-class explosions at various heights from 11km to 37km. Most occurred over the oceans and the only people killed were indirect victims drowned by resultant tsunami. No one suspected that the earth had been bombarded.

> Scenario H: 10 megaton-class explosions of which three were in excess of 25 megatons. These were 103, 83 and 27-megatons exploding at heights of 22km, 19km and 19km, respectively. In this 'century' there were massive casualties because one impact was over a populated part of Europe. No one on the planet remained in any doubt about hazards from space.

There is no need to go into more detail about Lewis' computer runs. It just needs to be stressed that Lewis is a serious astronomer using absolutely current data to work out likely century-impact scenarios, i.e. ask your friendly neighbourhood astronomer about the likelihood of impacts from space and this is what you get. These scary scenarios have to be compared with the answers you would get from most historians and archaeologists (there are no impacts in recent millennia apart from Tunguska, *assuming they have even heard of Tunguska*) and from 'asteroid astronomers' (there are no impacts and even Tunguska was a freak event of a sort unlikely to be repeated in millennia).

Going back to the Lewis scenarios, the important point is that back in time there were fewer people on the planet. There were vast uninhabited, or sparsely inhabited, areas, and communications and literacy were poor to non-existent over most of the planet. So failure to record impacts would have been the norm; something which we do indeed see in the historical record. Now, readers may balk at these last two statements, thinking 'Hold on, it could just as easily be the case that no historical record of impacts means there were no impacts'. Here the reader would be wrong. As Lewis pointed out, we know from many strands of evidence broadly what the impact rate should be over time. The fact that impacts are not in the historical record is *not* because none happened. After all, there are those well-attested crater fields that were formed in the last few millennia in Estonia, Poland, Germany and Italy – which were not recorded historically; their existence was deduced from holes in the ground. So we know the recording mechanism is flawed! What needs to be added from the Lewis scenarios is one key piece of intuitive thinking. Here is a quotation from his Scenario D:

(In this scenario) In 1946 a 25,000-metric-ton achondritic fireball explodes at 4:00 A.M. local time at a height of 11km above Fergana, Uzbekistan. The 1-megaton blast damages buildings over an area several kilometres in diameter, searing the area with intense heat and setting thousands of fires. The fires burn out of control, killing 4,146. Over 20,000 residents are awakened by a brilliant flash of light and heat to find their city in flames. An 'earthquake' is reported by the survivors. Several metric tons of meteorite fragments are mixed in with the debris of 2000 burned-out and collapsed buildings, where they are indistinguishable from scorched and blackened fragments of structural brick and rock.[3]

The important point that Lewis makes is this. If we go back in time there was no monitoring which would definitively allow the separation of an impact from an earthquake. This would be the case, especially, if the event were to take place in an earthquake-prone region. In his Scenario D there were no observations to link the disaster to its true cause. So even at the end of that particular century-long simulation run, no one suspected a hazard from space.

This is considerable food for thought. There are many earthquakes recorded in history. There are *no* impacts. Are we sure, given the spectre raised by Lewis, that all our historical earthquakes were *earth*-quakes. Worse still, we know from the Tunguska event that the ground shook out to a distance of 900km at the time of that aerial detonation. We can assume that in any major impact there will have been earth tremors. Survivors of such an event, who may have been some distance from the epicentre, may only have had a flash, an earth tremor, and a thunderous noise, to go on. If for any reason the flash was not observed, or even if it was, the survivor may only have reported an earthquake, just as Lewis suggests. Although this issue – that some earthquakes might actually be impacts – was raised in Chapter 7, there it was imagined that it would have been distant reporters who would have got things wrong, i.e. there was an impact and people, hundreds or thousands of kilometres away, only felt the earthquake; so only an earthquake was reported. What Lewis has done is raise the spectre that some well-known historical earthquakes – where perhaps a city was destroyed – were actually impacts that *were misreported* at the time. It has always been assumed that actual historical earthquakes – with levelled towns or cities – were just that, earthquakes. Now, thanks to Lewis, there is at least the freedom to question that comfortable assumption.

This point is so important that it deserves a little repetition. We inhabit a planet where the current wisdom is that the worst natural events we have to deal with are earthquakes and tsunami. History is littered with earthquakes, they kill people, but they are inherently local and we can live with them. They tend to occur mostly, though not exclusively, in earthquake zones. People who live in such areas accept the risk. People outside those areas have little need to worry. Now imagine that a percentage of recorded earthquakes were not tectonic in origin, but were in fact impact related. If that were the real situation then these events can take place anywhere; nowhere is safe. Suddenly, in this scenario, the whole world is a much scarier place. So, are there historical earthquakes which might actually have been impacts? One obvious possibility springs to mind, namely the great Antioch earthquake of AD 526. The writer John Malalas provides a strange description of the Antioch earthquake of 526. He talks of it as 'the fifth calamity from the wrath of God' and describes it as follows:

> ... those caught in the earth beneath the buildings were incinerated and sparks of fire appeared out of the air and burned everyone they struck like lightning. The surface of the earth boiled and foundations of buildings were struck by thunderbolts thrown up by the earthquakes and were burned to ashes by fire ... it was a tremendous and incredible marvel with fire belching out rain, rain falling from tremendous furnaces, flames dissolving into showers ... as a result Antioch became desolate ... in this terror up to 250,000 people perished.[4]

Now, one has to be careful with issues like this. There are other descriptions of the Antioch quake which lack the extreme 'colour' of this one. However, given the Lewis suggestion of impacts being mistaken for earthquakes, we should probably retain an open mind on whether this Antioch 'earthquake' might be an actual example of a misconstrued impact. After all, no one has ever searched for evidence of extraterrestrial material at Antioch – because it was just an earthquake? There is another example of such a destruction that also springs to mind. It relates to the events of the twelfth century BC that we saw in Chapter 5. In this Bronze

Age case, a bombardment event would actually help to explain the long-standing dilemma associated with the widespread destructions and burnings around the eastern Mediterranean in the twelfth century BC. Robert Drews set the scene well when he described what he termed 'the Catastrophe'. Here is what he said:

> ... the end of the Bronze Age was arguably the worst disaster in ancient history, even more calamitous than the collapse of the Western Roman Empire.[5]

It seems that many major sites were *totally destroyed* and *totally burned* at this time. The problem was (and is) that there were almost no bodies or precious objects. This evidence, coupled with Egyptian references to marauding hordes – the 'Sea Peoples', led to the assumption that the cities were destroyed by invaders who took away the inhabitants for slaves and carried off all the objects as booty before destroying and torching the cities. But that package actually creates a problem; almost by definition if no traces are left it is hard to prove that the invaders existed. Drews points out that there are other theories to explain 'the Catastrophe' involving concepts such as drought and 'system collapse', but he dismisses these in favour of the theory that the introduction of new slashing swords, and close-order fighting formations, allowed the 'invaders' to defeat everyone in the eastern Mediterranean and destroy and burn their cities. The problem as always seems to be that there ought to have been at least a few dead warriors and some weapons, but, by and large, there were not.

It was for that reason that other workers proposed that the widespread total destructions were actually caused by a huge earthquake storm.[6] Nice idea. Unfortunately it is almost unimaginable that you could have such severe earthquakes and not have lots of buried artefacts and people. What we seem to have here is a failure to recognise all the possible origins for destruction and fire. In the twelfth century BC the people probably still died in 'the Catastrophe', which, if it was extraterrestrial in character, would have involved destruction and fire from above. However, in all likelihood they would already have fled their towns and cities. This is because extraterrestrial events will often have precursor activity. For example a comet may be observed for some time before it comes close to the earth. Astronomers even recognise that a comet, or comet fragment, could in theory be captured into a short-term orbit before impacting the planet. If urban populations felt threatened there would be a tendency to flee the cities for the 'safety' of the countryside. With this sort of thinking we could explain all the phenomena relating to the twelfth-century BC destructions. This would include (i) the simultaneous destructions, (ii) the character of the destruction, (iii) the lack of bodies and, (iv) the strange distribution of artefacts. For example, Drews, talking of six major destroyed cities, points out that 'what gold, silver, and bronze items archaeologists found in these cities had been secreted in pits or hidden in wall caches.' This is reinforced by some relevant details from the site of Kokkinokremos in Cyprus where a bronze-smith put raw materials and tools into a pit while a silver-worker hid two silver ingots and a goldsmith hid his whole stock in another pit. Apparently 'they were all hoping ... that they would return and recover their treasures, but they never did.'[7]

It is this information, that the only valuables were hidden and never recovered, which suggests that the people who fled the cities were indeed killed. So the whole package – total abandonment, total destruction, total burning, hidden valuables, no one returning and the onset of a centuries-long dark age – would be entirely consistent with extraterrestrial bombardment. Ironically Drews came very close to this conclusion at one point. In discussing the unusual nature of the total destructions of the twelfth century, he wonders if they *were* actually due to an earthquake:

> Damage is one thing, however, and destruction is another. In all of antiquity only a few cities are known to have been destroyed by an 'act of God.' Whatever may have happened to Sodom and Gomorrah, we do know that Thera and Pompeii were covered by volcanic eruptions. And very occasionally we do hear of a city *destroyed* (rather than damaged) by an earthquake.[8]

Drews' best parallels for the total destruction which he surveyed in the eastern Mediterranean, in the twelfth century BC, were the very cities that had been destroyed when 'the Lord rained down brimstone and fire from heaven' upon them. It seems that there has to be a finite possibility that the twelfth-century catastrophe was caused by some extraterrestrial vector just as the Chinese mythical links suggest.

CONCLUSION

The issue of earthquakes and tsunami being secondary symptoms of impacts was raised speculatively in Chapter 7. With Lewis' additional input we can see that there is a real issue here. Some actual impact sites may have been misinterpreted as earthquakes! It is fair to say that no one has ever gone to the site of an ancient earthquake and searched it for debris of extraterrestrial origin. As a result, we do not know if any ancient earthquakes actually were due to impacts.

We have to remember that, in the current wisdom, the only impact from space that ever caused an earthquake was Tunguska in 1908. Does that sound likely; *that the only example of a particular phenomenon, in the whole of recorded history, took place in the last 100 years*? Simple statistics tell us how unlikely this is. There are 52 centuries of recorded history. Thus there is only one chance in 52 of any unique phenomenon occurring in a given century, i.e. the chance of Tunguska being unique (in the sense of occurring in 'our' century) is one in 52. Again, we could ask if there are any anomalous destructions in history. As indicated, destructions such as that at Antioch in the sixth century, and in the Mediterranean in the twelfth century BC, certainly exist, and there are many others. The possibility that some of these events might have been extraterrestrial in origin has never been tested.

This last sentence is interesting in itself. Absolutely everyone knows that in the past people feared comets. Given that fact, one would have thought that those studying the destructions of the twelfth century BC would at least have asked themselves the question 'Is it possible these destructions might have had something to do with comets?' But no, the question seems never to have been asked. 'Sea Peoples' and 'earthquakes' are the only games in town. Yet there was this traditional fear of comets. To ignore that traditional fear researchers must either have been assuming that people in the past were misguided, i.e. there were no grounds for the fear, or … what? Perhaps we should turn the question around. What was it that so successfully *stopped* people asking the question? The hints were certainly out there, whether in the form of the Sodom and Gomorrah story, the Phaethon myth, or in the quite specifically twelfth-century BC stories of the Battles of Troy, Mu, or Moytura. But, no one has ever acted on them and asked the question.

Well, actually, that is not true. Plenty of people *outside mainstream historical scholarship* have asked themselves whether comets might have been involved in ancient catastrophes. For example, the issue has been widely discussed among a worldwide brotherhood of what can best be described as 'retired engineers and librarians'.[9] However, they have been systematically ignored, marginalized or ridiculed; but mostly just ignored. Now writers like Lewis are laying the facts on the line. Now governments are funding Spaceguard-type programmes to monitor near-earth objects. Now NASA is sending spacecraft to intercept and study *both* asteroids and comets, with a view to deflecting anything that might threaten to hit the earth. Frankly, it is time for historians and archaeologists to wake up and start playing their part.

In case readers think this is simply rhetoric, this is as good a place as any to mention a forthcoming event. On 13 April 2029 an asteroid named Apophis will pass by the earth at a distance of less than 50,000km. If you're alive at the time, and it is not cloudy, you'll be able to see it pass with the naked eye. Apophis is more than 300m in diameter. If, as it passes the earth, it just happens to pass through a certain narrow window in space, then, in 2036 it will return and hit the earth (this narrow 'window' is a point where the earth's gravity would deflect the orbit of Apophis just enough to ensure an impact in 2036). Due to its mass, Apophis carries about 200 times the energy of the Tunguska object. If Apophis hits the earth the impact will be in the 3000-megaton class. It is entirely reasonable to state that such an impact, taking place anywhere on the planet, would collapse our current civilization and return the survivors, metaphorically speaking, to the Dark Ages (it is believed that in such an event globalised institutions, such as the financial and insurance markets, would collapse, bringing down the entire interconnected monetary, trade and transport systems). Impacts from space are not fiction, and it seems highly likely that quite a number have taken place in the last few millennia (over and above the small crater-forming examples already mentioned). It is just that, for some reason, most people who study the past have chosen to avoid, or ignore, the issue.

From this chapter we now know to suspect that not all recorded earthquakes were tectonic in origin, some will have been the secondary effects of impacts from space. Don't say you have not been warned.

THE 1290S SET THE TONE

Going back to the tree-ring story in Chapter 2, it was noticeable that, apart from the downturn in the 1340s, there was a highly coherent global tree-ring downturn in the early 1290s (*14* and *15*). Something pretty unpleasant took place in the years 1292-5 as far as trees were concerned. This short-lived downturn must have affected enormous numbers of trees to show up as clearly as this in a wide grid of chronologies from around the world. Subsequently, as information was accumulated, it became clear that around this time there was a cluster of references to fireballs from different areas. For example, the *Irish Annals* state that 'lightning and meteors destroyed the corn' in 1294.[1] This seemingly random observation takes on a little more significance when it is discovered that in 1295 '10 fireballs the size of houses' fell in China,[2] while there was a notable extraterrestrial impact in Russia, near Velikii Ustiug in 1296.[3] It appears that there was a distinct whiff of extraterrestrial bombardment during the decade.

Although it may seem like stretching the argument, there is a different sort of tree-ring event in the next year, 1297. Hughes and Brown working with sequoias (giant redwoods) from the American west coast, note that there is growth release – anomalously wide rings – after fire damage and they mention a very severe fire which caused this effect at their Mountain Home site in 1297. Sequoias are so large, and their wood is sufficiently fire resistant, that they are rarely killed by a low-level fire. However, they can record the fire in their ring record. This growth release in 1297 might not seem relevant at first sight. However, we know that one of the tree-ring phenomena noted after the explosion at Tunguska was growth release in many of the surviving trees (the growth release could be due to removal of competition and/or release of nutrients by burning). So this unusual fire in California in 1297 might sit comfortably with the list of fireball events in 1294-6.

SOME BACKGROUND ON THE ICE CORES

From Chapter 10 the reader now has some familiarity with the issue of the ammonium record from Greenland. However it may be worth setting out a bit more detail on the information that is available, before we embark on a more detailed analysis.

(i) The European GRIP core

The first record used was from the European GRIP ice core. It was at 55cm resolution and it was the one that showed large ammonium spikes at AD 539 and 1014. It is paralleled by a series of electrical conductivity (ECM) measurements that are useful for showing how much acid is present in the ice. High values in the ECM record tend to show up points where there is plenty of nitric or sulphuric acid. However, if there is a lot of ammonium in a particular layer it can serve to neutralize the acid with the result that we see anomalously low ECM values (such low ECM values are termed 'acid kills' for clarity). We shall see an example of this a little later. The GRIP ammonium record has two important advantages. First, the European workers did not lose any ice during the coring, so the 55cm sections are contiguous. Secondly, the dates associated with the individual sections are based on layer counting and in this the European ice-core workers have been helped enormously by having replicate cores. The three cores are known as Dye3, GRIP and NGRIP respectively. In fact due to the NGRIP corer breaking several hundred metres down, a second NGRIP core was taken, meaning that for the last two millennia there are actually four cores.

(ii) American GISP core:

The American GISP2 cores were taken only some 30km from the GRIP site at Summit, Greenland. The chemical records from the long GISP2 core (the 'deep core'), and from a shorter (GISP2 B) core, are both available.[4] The GISP2 core runs from 1985 back to the last interglacial, but for our purposes only the section that parallels the GRIP core back to 800 BC is of interest. It has to be stated that the GISP2 records are not so well replicated as the European cores, and further back in time the American workers lost sections of their long core. There is also a high-resolution GISP2 chemical record, but it is only available for limited periods, e.g. in the thirteenth-century data is provided for the years 1290-5, while for the fourteenth-century data covers 1316-20, 1356-62 and 1393-7.[5]

(iii) The Antarctic DomeC core:

There is another detailed electrical conductivity record from the DomeC ice core from Antarctica. Here again a little detail is required. The DomeC core is at high resolution, with measurements every 2cm.[6] While this is fantastic detail, the problem is that the dating is not quite so well constrained. For example,

DomeC being in Antarctica cannot be expected to have diagnostic Icelandic tephra layers to act as dating control. However, there may be a way around this particular problem. One key sulphate layer, observed in both Greenland and Antarctica, is the 1259 acid. In fact identical tephra has been found in the ice in both regions at this date, so it is likely that the volcano was somewhere close to the equator. This layer has been dated in three cores (Dye3, GRIP and GISP2) to 1259; so that is the working date. To get to the point, the large ECM signal relating to 1259 is actually dated in the DomeC core to around 1255.5, some 3.5 years too old. On the basis of this the acid-kill events in the thirteenth and fourteenth centuries in the DomeC record have been moved forward in time by three years, and it is these revised dates that are included in any succeeding tables.

In summary, the ice-core records form a rather disparate data set of various 'qualities'. However, as will become obvious, they represent a highly important source of information at close to annual, i.e. historical resolution. They tell us something of what was in the atmosphere in the past, when human populations were having their adventures. The question is can their records be integrated with the documentary record left by those humans who breathed that same atmosphere, but who only rarely commented on its quality?

A SHORT EXCURSION BACK TO SIXTH CENTURY

The reader knows, from Chapter 10, that for the years AD 1908, 1014, 626 and 539 ammonium in the GRIP ice record may well be the by-product of extraterrestrial bombardment by bolides or fireballs. We also know that research has its complications. For example, at 539 we have an acid kill simultaneous with the large ammonium spike (the acid in the ice having been neutralized, presumably by the ammonium). The question is can we always expect this to happen? It seems that we see the same thing at 626 because there is a reduction in conductivity in the Antarctic ice record at that date. However, at 1014 we seem not to have an acid kill even though at that date we have the *highest* ammonium value in two millennia. Then, to complicate matters, at 1908 there are notable amounts of chlorine, sulphate and nitrate at the same time as the big ammonium spike. This means that we cannot just read off a package of information in any simple way. However it is worth seeing what we have in the 1290s record.

Date	Fireballs etc.	GRIP	GISP 'B' Short core	GISP2 'D' core	DomeC (- 3Yr) Acid Kill
1290					
1291		1291.5 NH4	1291.4 NH4		
1292				1292.6 NH4+NO3	
1293			1293.0 NH4		
1294	Ireland 'lightning and meteors'			1294.8 NH4	Acid kill
1295	China 'fireballs'				Acid kill
1296	Russia 'fireball'	1296.7 NH4			Acid kill
1297					Acid kill
1298					
1299					

Table 1 Compilation *of* some historical information with chemistry from the GRIP, GISP2 and DomeC ice cores for the years 1290-99

With the ammonium records some caution is necessary. Each ammonium record in the GRIP core relates to a 55cm section of ice. This, in round figures, relates to a range of about 2.75 years (the ammonium could be concentrated anywhere in this 55cm length thus giving a bit of flexibility to the dating of the actual ammonium layer). The GISP2 chemistry should be correctly dated because the core records both sulphate and nitrate signals in the year 1362 which should be the known Öraefajokull eruption in Iceland. So let's talk our way through this table taking the results at face value.

In mid-1291 we seem to have replication between the GRIP and GISP2 cores, with both showing ammonium and GISP2 also showing nitrate. It cannot be impossible that it is this event that starts the poor growth seen in the global tree-ring curve. Then, in the years 1293-6 we see several ammonium and nitrate signals coinciding with historical records of meteors and fireballs, and accompanied by bad growth conditions for trees worldwide. An obvious question is where the ammonium, dated at 1296.7 in the GRIP core, actually occurs. If it were as early as early 1295 it might well replicate the 1294.6 nitrate layer in GISP2. As can be seen, this is a difficult game to play because of the limitations of chronology even at this refined level.

What we can say is that there seems to be a nitrogen-based package of events in the period 1291-7 that may hint at some high-energy material entering the atmosphere, consistent with the historical records of meteors and fireballs in 1294-6.

This coincides with several types of downturn and damage in tree-ring chronologies from around the world. Notice that there is no hint of sulphate in this mid-1290s episode, and that means we are probably entitled to rule out volcanic activity as the vector. With no evidence for volcanic activity, and with positive evidence for widespread meteor activity, it seems reasonable to link the ammonium, nitrate and acid-kill evidence to extraterrestrial bombardment.

BRITTON'S COMPILATION

C.E. Britton published his compilation of meteorological information back in 1937.[7] We now know things about the 1290s that he could not have been aware of. This seems like a good opportunity to look through Britton's compilation and see how it compares with our information. In this way we can judge whether his British and Irish information is reliable. Obviously if it is reliable it suggests that we might have reasonable confidence in similar information from the fourteenth century. This trawl through his list is not intended to be exhaustive. In addition, it is probably worth cautioning that, even in the late thirteenth century, there is often disagreement about exactly which year a document refers to. However this does not mean that we cannot get a flavour of the sort of records kept from the time. In the case of his first example we can use the reference to show that some of the evidence, that back in 1937 seemed obscure, can now be seen in a wider context, and can now be taken as substantiated.

First the example:

> On 18 July 1293 in central England there was 'a remarkable appearance in the sky about dawn' and the following evening there was 'continual thunder' for the whole night with great lightning, 'and finally there succeeded a thunderbolt'. Then just a year later, on 20 July 1294, 'there were coruscations of lightning destroying the corn whence ensued a great dearth and many died of hunger.[8]

In the past, references like this would have been ignored as irrelevant. However, we now know that 1293 and 1294 fall in a short, global, tree-ring downturn. We also know that there is ammonium in the ice cores at around this date. So, we are entitled to contemplate that the environmental downturn, as witnessed by the tree-rings, may have been the direct result of an extraterrestrial bombardment. Given that we know about the ammonium and about the various references to fireballs, we can take this entry in our stride

Britton looked at the same information and hazarded a guess that the two records were referring to the same event. If it was the same event, then we would not know in which year it occurred, 1293 or 1294. As noted above, the *Irish Annals* record that 'lightning and meteors destroyed the blades of corn' in 1294. Given the fuller account for 1293, and the replicated record for 1294, there seems no good reason to lump the 1293 and 1294 records together. The very fact that they are almost on the same day of the year could actually be consistent with the earth passing through the same stream of meteoric debris exactly one year later. It seems that we have 'a thunderbolt' and 'meteors' pretty certainly in 1293, with a reasonable possibility that there was something similar in 1294. There has to be the possibility that all the records are accurate, and that there were fireballs recorded in each of the years 1293-6; with a strong additional hint, because of the July dates, that this was enhanced Taurid activity.

Britton also found a reference to a terrible wind – an unusually severe wind – associated with what may have been an earthquake in January 1294 (which of course means January 1295). Here it seems reasonable to ask the following. If you are living in a period with regular bombardments from space, was the wind just wind, and was the earthquake just an earthquake? Or were these simply symptoms of a distant Tunguska-type explosion? But this very consideration raises an interesting issue. If the reader were to accept this re-interpretation, it would raise the spectre that some references to severe storms, or tempests, have been too easily ignored in the past. A storm is a storm and hence a mere meteorological phenomenon. But storms occur so regularly that if all storms were recorded they would swamp the whole record. In fact storms are referred to only sporadically. This implies that the *extreme terms* used about the storms that are recorded – 'tempests', 'whirlwinds' whatever – may actually be metaphors for more extreme events. Obviously it is not sensible to claim that every reference to a storm is a disguised reference to an impact. However, a few seemingly mundane descriptions from the past might, just might, be reasonable attempts to record real happenings that are not quite what they seem. The point being that Britton also found evidence from 1294 of continual rains in August and September. He found a shortage of wheat and severe famine. There was another 'prodigy' on 11 April and an extremely unusual fall – 'the grettest snowe that evere was seyn before this tyme'- on 14 May 1294 (although this, again, may have actually been in 1293). We could say 'it seems that this was an unsettled period for some reason.' In fact, of course, we are told the reason – the meteors are the reason – but we are mostly unwilling to accept what we are told. Should we be so unwilling? What is it that stops us accepting the references to meteors? The suspicion has to be that it is the derision heaped on us by colleagues, and the risk to employment prospects, that actually stops us accepting references to meteors as important. After all when these ancient records say that 'there was an earthquake', we accept that; when they say 'lightning struck a belfry', we accept that; what is it about records of meteors that is so unacceptable? The answer of course is that meteors are outside human control, and history is driven by people, not undisciplined natural events.

For the rest of the decade of the 1290s Britton found river floods, 'a great storm of hail snow and strong frost' affecting Scotland, violent windstorms, the sun the colour of blood. It seems reasonable to summarize the 1290s as 'unsettled' in common parlance. It clearly was not a benign period. However, all in all, the lesson we can draw is that the various statements all seem perfectly believable, and in the case of 1293 and 1294 they are well backed up by the independent testimony of the trees.

CONCLUSION

Readers may think that too much is being read into the scant evidence for goings-on in the 1290s. However, the decade has served to demonstrate a few points. There is a widespread tree-ring downturn that has never been commented upon before. There is a surprising cluster of references to meteors in the middle years of the decade. There is both ammonium and nitrate in the Greenland ice. Importantly, nothing recorded by Britton in his compilation of meteorological information seems unreasonable. There is nothing that sounds mythological or bizarre. The coincidence of an unusual wind with an earthquake is interesting when placed in the context of the cluster of observed meteors. In this sense the 1290s serve as a useful introduction to the fourteenth century. Overall, reading the information from the decade, suggests that the writers were doing their best to accurately describe what they were experiencing.

FOURTEENTH-CENTURY ICE
AND OTHER RECORDS

In this chapter a series of tables are presented bringing together the various ice core, and other, records for the fourteenth century. *Table 2* shows the main elements from 1300-15.

Date	Inundations Earthquakes (In : Eq)	GRIP	GISP 'B' Short core	GISP2 'D' core	DomeC (- 3Yr) Acid Kill
1300			1300.9 NH4		
1301	2xEq	1301.6 NH4			
1302		Acid kill			
1303	2xEq	Acid kill	1303.6 NH4		Acid Kill
1304		1304 NH4		1304.9 NH4	
1305					
1306				1306.7 NH4	
1307	In				
1308	Eq; In	NorthGRIP			
1309		NH4+AK			Acid Kill
1310		NH4+AK			Acid Kill
1311	Eq	NH4+AK			Acid Kill
1312					
1313	In				
1314	In				
1315					

Table 2 Compilation of some historical information with chemistry from the GRIP, GISP2 and DomeC ice cores for the years 1300-15

As noted before, because of the 55cm core problem, the ammonium layers in the GRIP core are dated only to a range of about 2.75 years. So, the two ammonium layers at 1301.6 and 1304 in that core could represent a *single* large event at the transition between the two 55cm sections, i.e. something at around 1303. Alternatively it could be that there are two separate signals, one in each section, e.g. one at 1301 and one at 1304. Without additional information it would not be easy to separate this issue. However, in this case we have the ECM record from the same core. Across 1300-5 in GRIP there is only *a single* ECM depletion (an acid kill). This suggests very strongly that the two high ammonium values are disguising one single very high value at around 1303 (the high ammonium neutralizing the acid signal). When added to the presence of ammonium in the GISP core it seems reasonable to suggest that somewhere in the period 1303-4 there was a quite significant ammonium event.

Table 2 also shows that there were two earthquakes recorded in 1303, but these were no ordinary earthquakes. A search around this period showed that there was a huge earthquake in China with its epicentre at Zhaocheng and Hongdong in Shanxi province. This quake took place on 25 September 1303 and is suggested to have been a 'scale 8' event. The language used speaks for itself: 'The 1303 earthquake havoc region has a major axis of 200km'.[1] The concept of a 'havoc region' the width of England is hard for westerners to come to terms with. Apparently more than 100,000 houses were damaged in the earthquake while 'mountains were destroyed and cities were removed .... Hongdong and Linfen were destroyed'. According to the same source 'more than 200 thousand people were pressed flat and several hundred thousand were injured'.[2]

One cannot help wondering if this was an example of Lewis' mistaken attribution. There is ammonium in the ice cores and we can hazard a guess that it was not produced by the earthquake. Would anyone have checked for extra-terrestrial debris in the region? Pretty certainly the answer to that question is 'no, it was a terrible *earthquake*'. In case the reader thinks too much is being read into this; in fact, nothing is being read into it. It is merely being pointed out that there is a coincidence between an ammonium spike and a major earthquake.

However, when we turn to the other 1303 earthquake we are confronted with an event that has puzzled even those who have studied it. It took place on 8 August, just seven weeks before the quake in China. It was felt strongly 'in Lower Egypt for about 15 min and caused widespread damage in Crete, Egypt, Rhodes, Jordan, Syria, Palestine, Turkey and Cyprus.'[3] This geographical spread and the details, such as the catastrophic effects in Crete, and the simultaneous effects in Egypt, hundreds of kilometres away (e.g. the bed of the Nile was exposed and boats were thrown onto the banks of the river), forced the authors, El-Sayed *et al.*, to come up with an intriguing notion. They reckoned that the best explanation was *two earthquakes on the same day.* One, in the Hellenic arc, would explain the 'observed tsunami and the extensive damage in Crete, Rhodes, etc'. While the other 'beneath the Nile valley' would explain the Nile effects, and the damage in Cairo and along the river.

So, in a short period in 1303 there were two well-separated major (major to the point of being exceptional) earthquakes, one of which is best explained as an unusual 'double'. This introduction of 'simultaneous events' as an explanation looks like a case of special pleading. When we see that special pleading is invoked to uphold the current earthquake paradigm, we are entitled to ask if there might be an alternative explanation for unusual simultaneous earthquakes. There is no doubt that a fragmenting bolide could provide an agency for such a simultaneous happening. Unfortunately there is no other information to allow a judgment to be made. However, this is a year when we would have to leave open at least the possibility of an impact, as hinted at by the ammonium. Of anecdotal interest, 1303 is generally taken to be the date when Giotto first inserted a 'comet' in place of the more normal 'star' into a Nativity painting. Conventional wisdom suggests that this insertion was inspired by the 1301 apparition of Halley's Comet.[4] However, there has to be at least the *possibility* that Giotto was actually inspired by a great fireball (or two) crossing the sky in 1303.

Table 2 also suggests another ammonium event in the time window 1309-11. In this case there is evidence for acid kill in both a Greenland and an Antarctic core. This hints that ammonium was comparatively widespread. Since it is unlikely that 'biomass burning' would affect both hemispheres at the same time, it is probably worth considering that this event might be related to bolide activity. Interestingly if we refer back to the tree-ring evidence from Chapter 2, *Figure 15* shows that the opposite behaviour of trees in the two hemispheres starts just around 1310; it is pretty certain that something must have triggered this opposite behaviour, the question is, what?

Moving on, in *Table 3* we see the ice-core evidence for things happening in the years 1316-31. This period includes the years of the Great Famine in Europe which can be loosely defined as 1316-22.[5] What is very evident is that across 1317-8 there is evidence of both ammonium and nitrate concentrations in three cores. Given that the GISP detailed record has two stratified layers there have to be two discrete incidents across these years. At this point it is worth going back to something in Chapter 7. There we saw an unusual earthquake 'felt throughout England' on 14 November 1318. In the GISP detailed core there is a sharp spike of both ammonium and nitrate in the ice dated to 1318.63-1318.71. This is not very far from the date of the earthquake. In fact, given that there always has to be at least a little slop on the ice-core dating, one is left wondering if that quake might actually have been the secondary effect of an impact.

If we wanted, we could even imagine that droplets of nitric acid could have provided condensation nuclei for the excessive rains that affected Europe in these years. Looking back over this period the 1317-8 episode does have everything.

Date	Inundations Earthquakes (In : Eq)	GRIP	GISP 'B' Short core	GISP2 'D' Deep core and/or Detailed core	DomeC (- 3Yr) Acid Kill
1316	In; Eq				
1317		NH4	NO3	NH4 + NO3	
1318	In; Eq		Low NH4 + NaCl	NH4 + NO3 + NaCl	
1319	In; Eq				
1320				NH4 + NO3	
1321	In; Eq		Acid Kill		
1322	In; Eq				Acid Kill
1323	2xEq				Acid Kill
1324	In				Acid Kill
1325	In				Acid Kill
1326					Acid Kill
1327		NH4			
1328	In		SO4	SO4	
1329			NH4		Acid Kill
1330	In				
1331	In				Acid Kill

Table 3 Compilation of some historical information with chemistry from the GRIP, GISP2 and DomeC ice cores for the years 1316-31

There is an earthquake and an inundation, there is ammonium and nitrate, and there is a replicated NaCl (sodium chloride = salt) signal. One wonders if there is anything against the idea of an impact over one of the world's oceans producing all of these effects. There does not appear to be any sulphate in the ice cores between 1300 and the replicated layer at 1328, so we can take it that there is no significant volcanic activity around 1318 to complicate the situation.

MOVING ON TO 1332-42

This next period, 1332-42 (*Table 4*) gives the impression of nothing much happening with respect to the ice record. Nothing stands out and there is no replicated signal apparent in the ice. This is despite the fact that it is the very time when the radiocarbon-calibration curve is going from enrichment to depletion around the 1330s. This is the time of cold sea-surface temperatures in the north Atlantic, the big downturn in bristlecone pine growth, and the start of the historical package of happenings in the run-up to the 1340s. This typifies the nature of speculative research. While it

Date	Inundations Earthquakes (In : Eq)	GRIP	GISP 'B' Short core	GISP2 'D' Deep core	DomeC (- 3Yr) Acid Kill
1332	In; Eq				
1333					
1334	In; Eq				Acid Kill
1335	In				Acid Kill
1336	In				
1337	In	Acid Kill			
1338	In		1338.5 NH4		
1339	In				
1340		Crète core			Acid Kill
1341	In; Eq	NO3			
1342	Eq	NO3	SO4		

Table 4 Compilation of some historical information with chemistry from the GRIP, GISP2, Crête and DomeC ice cores for the years 1332-42

would have been nice to see some hint of a causative agent for the 1333-34 changes, would we are forced to recognise that it is possible to have some quite significant regime changes without any obvious forcing factor visible in the available records.

CONCLUSION

In this chapter we have looked at the available information from 1300-42; the run-up to the plague decade. The dates that do stand out from this viewpoint relate to the happenings in 1303 and those at the time of the Great Famine, 1317-8. It is something of a surprise that nothing of importance is apparent around 1333, a date where we might have expected some radical activity. This highlights the fascination in dealing with the past. Take as an example, the events around 1014 (described in Chapter 10) were a surprise discovery. Previously there were no grounds for thinking that the Battle of Clontarf was anything other than an historical battle. Now, with ammonium, an inundation, and the reference to a cloud that killed a multitude, it may be necessary to take another look. The problem is that when evidence is anticipated – as it might reasonably be around 1333 – the past simply lets us down. It seems that it is not there to conform to our views; it is there only for us to try to understand.

However, this exercise shows that, as with the tree-ring chronologies, the ice cores are beginning to fill out an independent, historical-quality record of some of the things that were going on in the world in the early-fourteenth century.

14

THE PLAGUE DECADE

Following on from 1342, in the run-up to the arrival of plague, we start to see something rather different to the patchy goings on in the previous decades. In *Table 5* all the available ice records for 1343-9 are laid out at higher resolution, with the whole range of dating estimates as given by the ice-core workers included. What we see is a consistent volcanic signal, including sulphate and enhanced electrical conductivity across 1344. Zielinski *et al.* reported a volcano in 1344 in their analysis of the GISP2 core.[1] This is pretty certainly the same sulphate layer that shows up in the GISP2 B core between 1341.2 and 1343.2 and in the Crête ice core in 1345.

There is also a volcanic event at 1344 in the Plateau Remote ice core in East Antarctica,[2] and, if the 3.5-year re-dating of the DomeC ice core is valid, it also shows up in this Antarctic core as a high-conductivity acid signal. That is pretty impressive consistency across ice cores from two hemispheres. Thus, the 1340s get off to a flying start with an unequivocal volcanic event. Though, interestingly, none of the ice-core workers single this particular acid layer out as significant in any way.

What we can see from *Table 5* is that, following the 1343-4 volcanic event, there is a clear and well-replicated pulse of ammonium *and* nitrate across almost all of 1345 and 1346. The stratigraphy of the ice means that this replicated layer of ammonium and nitrate is definitely *after* the 1343-4 sulphate layer. Obviously there may be a little flexibility in the exact specification of the dates (by perhaps a few months) but that does not affect the order of the events. The question, again, is what causes a consistent presence of ammonium and nitrate? Is this an example of a major forest fire (biomass burning) episode or is it impact-related, after the manner of Tunguska?

What is most striking about *Table 5* is the set of ammonium measurements spanning essentially the whole of 1347 and 1348. Again, these are stratigraphically *after* the ammonium-plus-nitrate package of 1345 and 1346. The dates from the cores are remarkably consistent, and there is every reason to believe (with the anchor of the 1362 Öraefajokull tephra) that they are calendrically precise.

Date	NGRIP Greenland	Plateau Remote Greenland	GRIP Greenland	GISP2 'B' Greenland	GISP2 'D' Greenland	DomeC-3 Antarctica	Summary
1343.7					SO_4	Acid	Volcano
1343.9					SO_4	Acid	Volcano
1344.1		SO_4	NH_4		SO_4	Acid	Volcano
1344.3		SO_4	NH_4		SO_4	Acid	Volcano
1344.5		SO_4	NH_4		SO_4	Acid	Volcano
1344.7		SO_4	NH_4		SO_4	Acid	Volcano
1344.9		SO_4	NH_4		SO_4	Acid	Volcano
1345.1			NH_4		SO_4	Acid	Volcano
1345.3			NH_4	NH_4+NO_3	SO_4		
1345.5			NH_4	NH_4+NO_3	NH_4+NO_3		NH_4+NO_3
1345.7			NH_4	NH_4+NO_3	NH_4+NO_3		NH_4+NO_3
1345.9			NH_4	NH_4+NO_3	NH_4+NO_3		NH_4+NO_3
1346.1			NH_4	NH_4+NO_3	NH_4+NO_3		NH_4+NO_3
1346.3			NH_4	NH_4+NO_3	NH_4+NO_3		NH_4+NO_3
1346.5			NH_4	NH_4+NO_3	NH_4+NO_3		NH_4+NO_3
1346.7			NH_4	NH_4+NO_3	NH_4+NO_3		NH_4+NO_3
1346.9					NH_4+NO_3		
1347.1			NH_4	NH_4	NH_4	Acid kill	NH_4+acid kill
1347.3			NH_4	NH_4	NH_4	Acid kill	NH_4+acid kill
1347.5			NH_4	NH_4	NH_4	Acid kill	NH_4+acid kill
1347.7			NH_4	NH_4	NH_4	Acid kill	NH_4+acid kill
1347.9			NH_4	NH_4	NH_4	Acid kill	NH_4+acid kill
1348.1	NH_4+acid kill	*QUAKE*	NH_4	NH_4	NH_4	Acid kill	NH_4+acid kill
1348.3	NH_4+acid kill		NH_4	NH_4	NH_4	Acid kill	NH_4+acid kill
1348.5	NH_4+acid kill		NH_4	NH_4	NH_4	Acid kill	NH_4+acid kill
1348.7	NH_4+acid kill		NH_4	NH_4	NH_4	Acid kill	NH_4+acid kill
1348.9	NH_4+acid kill		NH_4	NH_4	NH_4	Acid kill	NH_4+acid kill
1349.1			NH_4	NH_4	NH_4		
1349.3					NH_4		

Table 5 Detailed record (note time running from top to bottom of the Table) of chemistry from six ice cores acros 1344-48 showing the 1344 volcanic event and the concentration of ammonium across January 1348; the St Paul's Day earthquake is indicated

Here again it is necessary to caution the reader. The dates given for the sulphate, nitrate and ammonium all suffer from the 55cm curse, wherein the actual chemical signature does not have to be spread through the whole of the section of ice core. Thus, the 1343-4 sulphate layer merely has to be *somewhere* in 1343-4. It could in reality occupy only a few months of this two-year period (it is reasonable to think of the wider two-year spread as the 'error' on the dating). The same can be said for the ammonium-plus-nitrate layer which occurs in 1345-6. The actual layer is merely somewhere in the time-span 1345-6. Exactly the same applies to the 1347-8 ammonium layer; it does not have to span the whole of those two years, it could occur anywhere within the time-span.

What is critically important is the relationship of the ammonium to the 25 January 1348 earthquake. It could be that the ammonium was around either just before, or just after, or indeed right across, the time of the earthquake. One is free to wonder if the ammonium was due to an impact and whether, or not, it was actually produced on the same day. What the ice-core workers have done, by producing these several ammonium records, is raise the *possibility* that the fourteenth-century writer (who said that in his view the corruption of the atmosphere came from the earthquake of St Paul's Day, 1348) was actually correct. Here is scientific evidence for a corrupting gas being present in the earth's atmosphere within, at most, a few months of the specified date.

This survey of the ice-core results has a revelation-like quality. The reader has to remember that this evidence simply did not exist before. All of the deliberations about the use of the term 'corrupted atmosphere' over the last two centuries have been based on a variety of pre-suppositions. The principal one being that 'misguided' people in the past had 'wrongly' blamed plague on 'corrupted atmosphere'. Now we have real evidence that may show a genuine corrupted atmosphere right at the time of the Black Death. The question is: 'where did the ammonium come from; was it extraterrestrial in origin?' A second and equally important question must be: 'what else was in the atmosphere?'

This is a critical issue. It is widely assumed that the ice cores have undergone something approaching a *total* analysis. This is absolutely not the case; the analysis of the ice has never been exhaustive, we only have records of a few chosen chemicals. We do not know everything that is in the ice. There has to be the possibility that the ammonium simply represents the tip of an atmospheric chemical 'iceberg'. *Appendix 2* contains recent information on the chemical make up of comets. Ammonium is only one of a list of constituent chemicals that have now been identified. Some of the others are organic, particularly poly-aromatic-hydrocarbons. It is alarming to think what effect a whiff of some of this extraterrestrial chemistry might have had if humans were subjected to it.

Turning to anecdotal information, the Hecker/Ziegler compilation does provide us with '1343-47 assorted earthquakes, deluges, inundations and subterraneous thunder'. These could include secondary symptoms of volcanic activity in 1343-4, but equally they could be related to secondary effects of impacts from space. When the whole package across the 1340s is considered, it suggests, yet again, that there may be some scientific support for the contemporary fourteenth-century records.

CONCLUSION

Let us think of the ammonium/impact/plague scenario as a little scientific experiment. In the list of ammonium measurements for the current era (AD 1–1642) in the GRIP core there are 614 individual observations. Of these 614 observations there are 82 that have values *greater than 10 units of ammonium*. That means that one observation in every 7.5 observations has notably high ammonium. Let's now go through the ammonium dates relevant to the plague issue.

For the 540 event the closest ammonium value is at 539, a date which actually spans the calendar year 540 (because each ammonium measurement represents two to three years of ice). Plague arrives into continental Europe in 1348. We now know that there is a heightened ammonium value in four ice cores in 1348. To get a feel for how unlikely it would be to find enhanced ammonium at exactly those two dates we can simply multiply 7.5 by 7.5. The chance of finding enhanced ammonium at the exact start of the two greatest plagues in the last two millennia is about '1 chance in 56'. This fact, in itself, would constitute grounds for suspecting that there is a relationship of some sort between the occurrence of ammonium and the occurrence of plague. The relationship could of course be 'indirect', i.e. again the ammonium might just be a signpost for a package of unpleasant chemicals.

Perhaps curiously, Britton refers to a record relating to this same year:

> 1348 Lowe refers to 'dry fog with earthquake'. This somewhat cryptic entry does not seem to be supported by any reference to an early authority. No original record has been traced.[3]

It would seem from his tone that all the 'corrupted atmosphere' references had somehow passed Britton by. However 'dry fog' has a particular relevance. It refers specifically to a high-level loading of the atmosphere, such as was observed in 536-7 just before the arrival of the plague of Justinian's time. It would be intriguing to know what Lowe's source was. It does however leave us with references to 'dry fogs' – that seem not to be volcanic in origin – close to the dates of the two greatest plagues in the last two millennia, both marked by the presence of ammonium in Greenland.

COMET FREQUENCIES

The reader could be forgiven for thinking that this story about ammonium and impacts is a bit fanciful. If it was true surely astronomers would know about it already. The answer to that is, 'probably not'. After all, the conventional wisdom has been that ammonium is the product of forest fires. Almost the only clue that the ammonium in the ice cores might *not* be due to forest fires resides in the question marks in the titles of the relevant papers.[1] No one has been discussing ammonium and impacts, despite the suspicious occurrence of ammonium in mid-1908. Moreover, the increasingly narrow focus of most research means that there is little cross-fertilization across disciplines. Why would an astronomer know much of ice-core work, other than when the ice records indicate something about Milankovich orbital cycles, or extraterrestrial dust during ice ages? So, is there any way that direct astronomical observations can be linked to the observations of ammonium at 539 and 1348? We should note that there is the potential for a great prize here. If even a few ammonium spikes in the ice could be shown to be impact related it would open up a whole new research area on impact frequencies. Surprisingly, there is some information on historical observations that might just link into these two dates.

David Hughes recently took a detailed look at the history of the observation of long-period comets (long-period comets are those with periods of more than 200 years). His study revealed a number of points which most casual observers might miss. For example, in his abstract he says:

> The acuity of northern hemisphere naked-eye observers throughout the era of pre-telescopic astronomy was such that they were capable of observing 0.903+/- 0.088 long-period comets per year. This rate was not achieved in practise, but the combined efforts of Chinese, Japanese, Korean, Middle Eastern, European and North African observers got fairly close between AD 1355 and AD 1600.[2]

From the point of view of this book one is immediately struck by his use of the 1355 date. Did something change around the middle of the fourteenth century? Indeed it did. *Figure 32* shows the discovery rate of long-period comets (i.e. those with a period in excess of 200 years) for the period AD 400–1750. We should note that Hughes chose 1750 as a cut-off date because it marks the time around which interest in the predicted return of Halley's comet (in 1757) caused people to start systematically looking for comets; after 1750 the number of comet observations increases dramatically, aided by telescopic searches; previously all comet observations had been accidental.

Hughes produced this figure and obviously commented on the clear change of slope of the observations in the fourteenth century. He says:

> … between AD 1 and about AD 1330+/-40 the cumulative comet number increased
> steadily at the rate of 0.272 comets per year, 364 comets being recorded in this time

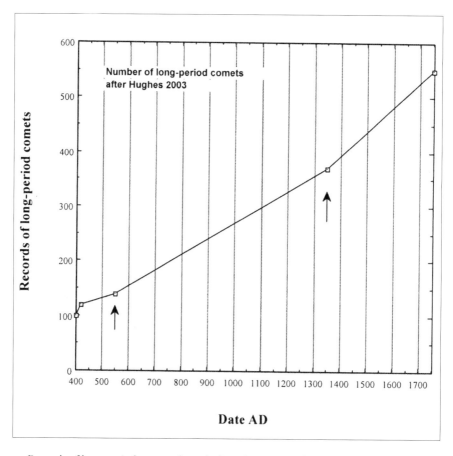

32 Records of long-period comets through time showing Hughes' changes in discovery rates around AD 550 and 1350. *After Hughes 2003*

interval. Between AD 1340 and AD 1750 the rate leapt to 0.466 per year, 191 comets being recorded in these 410 years.[3]

There is no need to re-argue Hughes' thesis here, rather it needs to be mined for information. For example, he says that between 100 BC and AD 1 there was only one comet recorded by both eastern and western observers (presumably the comet of 44 BC). Again, only one comet was observed between AD 200 and 300. It seemed to Hughes that, when it came to recording comets, the pre-AD 500 data was neither as complete, nor as reliable, as the AD 500-1700 data. The reader should by now be sensitized to such a statement. Something changed with respect to comet observations around *both* AD 500 and 1350!

One obvious possibility is that, at around these two dates, interest in comets altered. In both cases observations increased; observers clearly paying more attention to comets after these two dates. Yet these dates sit close to the two great plagues of the present era. That fact alone should trigger the question – did the plagues have something to do with comets? We now know that there was ammonium in the atmosphere at both these times and it is possible to argue a reasonable case that the ammonium could have had an extraterrestrial source. Does this imply that the increased interest in comets was *because they were associated in the minds of observers with corruption of the atmosphere* – exactly as tradition said? With this logic we are immediately thrown back to the ideas of Hoyle and Wickramasinghe. They have argued that diseases come from space, indeed, specifically from comets. We can now see that at least one medieval writer suggested that *pestilentia* meant 'the time of tempest caused by light from the stars'. Now we see that people observed more comets after the two great plagues. It makes a kind of sense.

There could, of course, be another explanation. It could be that after AD 500 there really were more comets, and again, after the 1340s there were still more comets. How could that be? Easily enough! If there were *fragmentations of comets* at around these two dates then we might reasonably expect more comets to be observed after each fragmentation.

All of this raises questions about what it was people in the past observed about comets and also how they recorded what they observed. If we go back to Hughes we find that his comments about comets all relate to long-period comets. Hughes points out that short-period (period less than 20 years) and intermediate-period (period between 20 and 200 years) comets are under-represented in the records. He actually says:

Only one short-period comet was seen before 1757, this being 6P/1678 R1 d'Arrest [period 6.6 years] …. Only three intermediate-period comets were discovered prior to 1757. 1P/Halley [period 76 years] … 55P/Tempel-Tuttle [period 33.4 years] … [and] … 109/P Swift-Tuttle [period 131 years].[4]

This comes as a real surprise. We have to believe that short-period comets were hardly being recorded in the past – how strange. However, there was something that Hughes could not know about past observations of short-period comets because it was buried in mythology!

THE MYTHICAL CONTEXT FOR SHORT–PERIOD COMETS

The reader has been exposed to several well-dated examples of myths and metaphors that genuinely do seem to be disguised descriptions of catastrophic happenings, and their causes. When Hughes' comment about the under-representation of short- and intermediate-period comets was noted, it resonated with some information contained in a recent book about Irish mythology, written with Patrick McCafferty. In that book we pointed out that many of the descriptions of the Irish gods/heroes, such as Lugh and Cúchulainn, bear remarkable similarities to comets drawn by nineteenth-century astronomers (while observing 'through the telescope').[5] What had struck us in particular were the curious gestation periods attributed to some of these 'mythical' characters. Here is how the Irish king Conchobar was conceived:

> Nes, the daughter of Eochaid Sálbuide of the yellow heel was sitting outside Emain with her royal women around her. The druid Cathbad from the Tratraige of Mag Inis passed by, and the girl said to him: 'What is the present hour lucky for?' 'For begetting a king on a queen', he said. The queen asked him if that were really true, and the druid swore by god that it was: 'A son conceived at that hour would be heard of in Ireland for ever'. The girl saw no other male near, and she took him inside with her. She grew heavy with a child. It was in her womb for three years and three months. And at the feast of Othar she was delivered.[6]

A multiple of this same peculiar gestation period is mentioned in another story:

> Fingel, who was to be the mother of Noidhiu Nae-mBreathach, was closely guarded lest anyone should make her conceive, but she was visited by a phantom from over the sea and was pregnant for nine months and nine years.[7]

So, although there are no observations of Comet Encke (the comet with the shortest period of just 3.3 years) in the historical record, people in Ireland in the first millennium AD seem to have been aware of the peculiar interval of three years and three months and were incorporating it into stories about the birth of heroes. The most reasonable assumption would be that people were aware of the return time of Encke but were incorporating its periodic returns into myth rather than recording it as a scientific observation (it is curious to note that, while Encke's period is 3.3 years, two of the four short- or intermediate-period comets that Hughes cites have periods of 6.6 and 33.4 years; twice and 10 times the period of Encke respectively).

Intriguingly, in Chinese myth the character No Chia (who we have already met in Chapters 5 and 10, and who belongs to a time more than a millennium earlier – traditionally twelfth century BC) was in his mother's womb for three years and six months. No Chia's ancestry goes like this:

> The eldest daughter of the Lord of Heaven had married the general Li Ching .... But before No Chia was born his mother had been carrying him for three years and six months.[8]

In the story, the mother was impregnated by a Taoist priest in a dream. In the dream the priest placed a brilliant pear inside her, and, on waking, she gave birth to 'a ball of flesh which spun like a wheel, filling the chamber with strange perfumes and red light'. This startled Li Ching and he cut the sphere in two with his sword revealing 'a small boy whose whole body glowed with a rosy radiance. His face was delicate and as white as snow'. This was No Chia. The father Li Ching was no ordinary mortal. The following is written about him:

> Li Ching, the pagoda-bearing king of heaven may perhaps be traced back to the god of thunder and lightning, Indra. The pagoda might then be a misinterpretation of the thunderbolt Vadira.[9]

So, the simple act of noting that several myths have peculiar time intervals (that are suspiciously close to the period of a comet) leads to characters which, in the Chinese case, are related to the king of heaven and his wife, the eldest daughter of the lord of heaven. Readers may be wondering just where this discussion is going. In fact, it leads somewhere quite profound. Note how in this strange myth, No Chia's parents sound remarkably closely related, as if the mother is both the wife and the sister of Li Ching, and No Chia has both a strange conception and a strange birth. If we turn to Welsh myth we can find a story about the birth of Lugh (the Celtic comet god we saw in Chapters 5 and 6) who in Wales is known as Lleu.

> Gwydion ... had also a sister Arianrhod or 'Silver Circle', who, as is common in mythologies was not only his sister but also his wife .... Of this connection two sons were born at one birth - Dylan and Lleu.[10]

Here we have Arianrhod, whose name means 'silver disc' or 'wheel' and whose place is in the sky – the constellation Corona Borealis is known as Caer Arianrhod, or Arianrhod's castle – giving birth to her sons by her husband who was also her brother:[11]

> Then she (Arianrhod) stepped over the magic wand, and with that step she dropped a fine boy-child with rich yellow hair. The boy uttered a loud cry. After the boy's cry she made for the door, and thereupon dropped a small something [*an 'afterbirth'*], and before anyone could get a second glimpse of it, Gwydion took it and wrapped a sheet of silk around it and hid it … inside a small chest at the foot of his bed …. As Gwydion was one day in his bed … he heard a cry in the chest … and as he opened it he could see an infant boy thrusting his arms from the fold of the sheet and opening it apart. (This author's italics.)[12]

So, in this story Arianrhod gives birth to a 'small something': a shapeless lump/an afterbirth that contained the 'hero' who was to be known as Lleu Llaw Gyffes (meaning 'bright – with a sure hand'). This is why it has always been accepted that the Lleu in Welsh myth is the same as Lugh Lamfhada (meaning 'bright – of the long arm').

Putting these stories together, in China we have No Chia whose mother and father are related to the lord/king of heaven; No Chia has a peculiar 3.5-year gestation period, and a most peculiar birth where he appears enclosed in a ball of flesh. In the Celtic west we have Lleu (Lugh) who is born as a 'small something': a shapeless lump, a kind of afterbirth. The question is can we find a link from Lugh to Conchobar, who also has that strange three year and three month gestation period? Well, yes we can. The Ulster god/hero Cúchulainn acts as a suitable link. Cúchulainn's mother is Dechtire (the sister of Conchobar), his father is Lugh and Conchobar is his uncle. So we can find a direct linkage from Conchobar to Lugh in the Irish stories – Lugh is Conchobar's son-in-law. This means that on opposite sides of the Old World there are stories about characters with similar, but very unusual, gestation periods. The stories then allow, in both cases, links to surprisingly similar strange births. The only logical explanation for this common linkage is that both sets of stories are recording similar goings on observed in the sky (specifically something breaking up – giving birth to an offspring - in the sky).

For readers not familiar with myth, the above is another good example of the way myth operates. These were important pieces of information to the ancient human witnesses of, in this case, powerful events in the sky. In pre-literate societies, e.g. in pre-Christian Ireland, the information was compressed and disseminated among people who knew the basic story. Storytellers could decompress the stories and tell them at greater length. The stories survived for long periods, but, somewhere along the way – either by people moving, or undergoing culture change, or forgetting, or no longer believing – the real meaning of the stories was lost. The stories to our modern, literate, ears appear to be gobbledegook, with bizarre people doing bizarre things – fairy stories. In point of fact, it is the stranger aspects that act as clues to at least partial decipherment of the myths. For example, when a god flies rapidly over both land and sea it is pretty clear that he is in the sky; when Arianrhod's castle is in the sky it is clear that she is not a flesh and blood princess; when a hero has a totally unnatural gestation period he is more likely to be a comet than a mere knight.

As noted earlier, both Lugh and Cúchulainn appear to be comet gods. In fact it is normally stated that Cúchulainn is not just the son of Lugh, he is the *rebirth* of Lugh, i.e. 'Lugh back again'. This is a very suitable relationship for a comet.

CONCLUSION

This chapter draws out an important point. If attempts are made to understand happenings in the fourteenth century solely by *looking back from the present*, across the quiescent centuries from 1400-2000, then the wrong perspective is being used. In earlier times there were catastrophic events at times when comets were recorded. However, those records have somehow become disconnected, in that no one now believes that the comets had anything to do with the catastrophic events. It seems that it is myth and metaphor that make the connection. Now we have even seen that short-period comets, that astronomers had assumed were *not recorded*, actually were recorded but in mythology not history.

How can this be summed up? In the past comets were feared, everyone knows that. They were sometimes recorded as plain text observations. On other occasions they were observed but were only recorded tangentially, in myth and metaphor. Either way, in recent times, references to them tend to be treated either with disbelief or dismissively, i.e. 'there may be references to a comet but it would not have had any effect on the ground'. So, when Ziegler says:

> The fact that the title 'Black Death' was not used by contemporaries similarly makes it hard to credit those other explanations which attributed the name to a black comet seen before the arrival of the plague.[13]

It is clear that he gives no weight to the fact that someone claimed to have seen a black comet before the plague arrived. Viewed from today, when comets seem to be distant, harmless, puffy, snowballs, his stance is probably correct. Viewed from the poorly understood 'total destructions' of the twelfth century BC, or the globally catastrophic environmental episode at the start of the Justinian plague, where myth and metaphor suggest that comets were the prime cause, his stance is probably wrong. The fact that someone once said 'a black comet was seen before the arrival of the Black Death' has now – post ammonium, post myth, post metaphor – to be seen as potentially important. Was it a comet so close that its jet-black, tarry surface could be seen by the naked eye? Was it a comet trailing a black organic dust tail? It would be important to know. If Roger of Wendover's 'vast comet seen from Gaul' was in all probability real, and probably caused the plague of 540, then why should not Ziegler's 'black comet' have been every bit as real, and why should not it have caused the Black Death; as someone at the time seems to have suggested. Perhaps it is as simple as this: when comets were far from the earth moving slowly across the sky over days or weeks they were recorded as comets. However, when a comet came close to the earth travelling at high velocity and presenting an astonishing aspect as it passed, perhaps it was not at all obvious what it was. This would be the case especially if it was too bright to look at; if electrophonic effects made it audible; and if it was delivering exploding fireballs into the atmosphere.

By specifying dates around the time of the two great plagues, when the rate of comet sightings/recordings increased, Hughes has provided a whole new perspective. This essentially closed loop makes perfect sense. Populations subjected to horrendous death rates may have felt they had good reason to be fearful of comets. If they related the comets to the corruption of the atmosphere then we can see why an increased awareness of comets would be an inevitable outcome. It is probably no accident that Gibbon commented on 'the atmosphere being corrupted' in the sixth century,[14] and Ziegler pointed out the widespread notion of the atmosphere being corrupted in the fourteenth century.[15]

We can now see that stories from Ireland to China almost certainly preserve information about the returns of Comet Encke (or possibly some sister comet with similar orbital characteristics, now extinct) and its decreasing period, from 3.5-3.3 years over the centuries from the twelfth century BC to the laying down of the Irish stories. Something even the astronomers had missed.

FURTHER ELABORATION
ON AMMONIUM

The idea of plague being associated in some way with ammonium is so important that it requires some additional support. One way forward is to elaborate on the ice records that provided the information in the first place. What follows will show that the ammonium scenario stands up to quite a reasonable degree of scrutiny. Here is what the interested reader needs to know.

We can demonstrate that the GISP2 core is consistent with the GRIP core back to around AD 1030 by plotting the two independent ammonium records. *Figure 33* shows a plot where each data set has been 'five-point smoothed'. This is a simple manipulation which slightly broadens the peaks in the data to take account of the bi-annual sampling of the ice. It is clear from *Figure 33* that across this period the two cores are in close agreement back to the middle of the eleventh century. We can therefore take it that the ammonium spikes at dates such as 1303 and 1348 really are replicated observations.

However, as we start to go further back in time, certainly by 1014, we start to see the GRIP and GISP2 records diverging. At this point we have to remember that the European GRIP core was continuous, whereas the GISP2 core had several 'lost' sections. At several places, most notably in the later sixth century (but also in the fourth century), sections of the American long core were 'trashed', i.e. when brought to the surface some of the 2.2m sections of core tended to 'explode' into ice cubes, due to internal pressure within the ice. These trashed sections inevitably introduce slight doubts concerning the chronological integrity of the GISP2 record.

When we look at the plot of the two smoothed records before 1030 the GRIP and GISP2 records *do not agree visually* when they are lined up using the dates provided by the ice-core workers. *Figure 34* shows the lack of agreement between the raw records. However, as dendrochronologists are used to matching time-series patterns, the smoothed records were compared visually and good agreement was observed, from around AD 750 to around 400 BC, *when the two records are displaced*

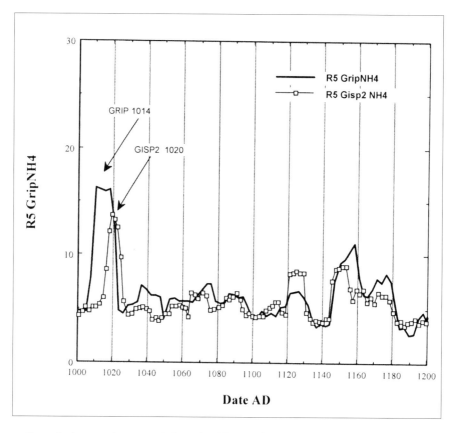

33 Smoothed ammonium records from the GRIP and GISP2 ice cores showing good agreement that starts to break down in the early eleventh century. *Data obtained from: The Greenland Summit Ice Cores CD-ROM. 1997[1]. Available from the National Snow and Ice Data Center, University of Colorado at Boulder, and the World Data Center-A for Paleoclimatology, National Geophysical Data Center, Boulder, Colorado*

by around 19 years. Figure 35 shows the much better agreement if the GISP2 core is lengthened by 19 years, i.e. if all the GISP2 dates older than AD 750 are moved back in time by 19 years.

One obvious question is why the GISP2 core should be moved rather than the GRIP core, in order to establish the 19-year revision? The answer to that relies purely on the fact that the European workers have three cores Dye3, GRIP and NGRIP (in fact 4 cores, because a duplicate NGRIP core had to be drilled). With this level of replication it is very unlikely that they could have missed any significant discrepancy. The GISP2 core, on the other hand, is a single core and its chronological consistency depends on the integrity of the layer-counting process. On balance, the offset between the two cores can best be explained by the American team counting about 19 layers *too few* in the two centuries between AD 1030 and 750.

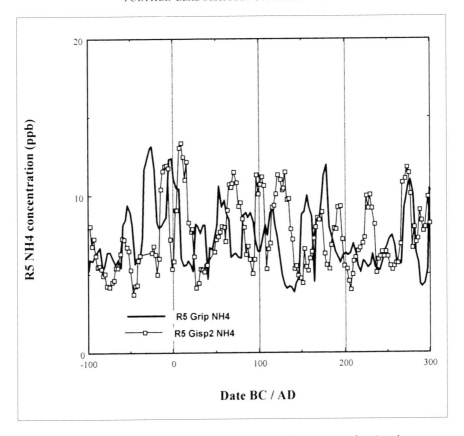

34 Smoothed ammonium records from the GRIP and GISP2 ice cores showing the poor agreement at the dates given by the respective ice-core groups. *Data obtained from: The Greenland Summit Ice Cores CD-ROM. 1997. Available from the National Snow and Ice Data Center, University of Colorado at Boulder, and the World Data Center-A for Paleoclimatology, National Geophysical Data Center, Boulder, Colorado*

Could such a thing happen? This is an interesting philosophical question. It depends on the parameters being used to distinguish individual annual layers in the ice cores. Normally there is a clear annual character to the profiles of dust and acidity. However, sometimes there can be internal structure to the annual profiles and this could lead to misidentification of real annual bands as internal structure within bands. It seems that this is what happened with the GISP2 core. Now, interestingly, although this proposed 19-year shift was deduced purely by looking at the two ammonium records, something very similar had already been independently suggested by John Southon based on the oxygen isotope records in the two cores. Although Southon was more interested in disagreements between the records further back in time, he did point out that:

GRIP data shifted by -20yr [i.e., to younger ages] fit the GISP2 results reasonably well over most of the period 1800-2500yr B.P.[2]

As already pointed out, it would seem more sensible to shift the poorly replicated, and incomplete, GISP2 record back in time by about 20 years rather than shift the well-replicated GRIP record. However, any way this is viewed, Southon's suggestion is exactly in line with the suggestion being made here with respect to the ammonium records.

THE GISP2 RECORD FROM AD 750-1050

It is possible to show how the two ice records can be reconciled. It is evident from *Figure 33* that the records agree well back to around 1030. If we accept that the Dye3, GRIP and NGRIP cores are correctly dated, then the large ammo-

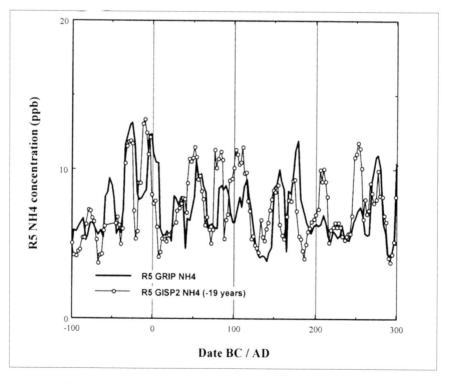

35 Smoothed ammonium records from the GRIP and GISP2 ice cores showing the improved agreement when the GISP2 record before AD 750 is *shifted back* by 19 years. *Data obtained from: The Greenland Summit Ice Cores CD-ROM. 1997. Available from the National Snow and Ice Data Center, University of Colorado at Boulder, and the World Data Center-A for Paleoclimatology, National Geophysical Data Center, Boulder, Colorado*

nium spike centred on 1014 in the European records is already about six years *too young* in the GISP2 record (for the purist, expressions like 'too young' are subjective; technically it might be more accurate to say that by 1014 the GISP2 core has lost about six annual layers and the record is about six years too short by that date). This implies very strongly that the American ice-core workers were already losing years from their counts of annual layers by the early eleventh century. As a partial check on this, we know that there is a major *sulphate* spike at 938 in the GISP2 core, a spike which is dated to 932 in Dye3 and to 934 in GRIP. Thus, the sulphate record also suggests that by the 930s GISP2 is about 4-6 years too short.[3] Following through this logic of comparing the ammonium records visually, we can justify inserting 6 years around 1030, another six years at 865 and a further seven years at 760.

Figure 36 shows the GRIP and GISP2 records plotted across AD 700-1050 with these cumulative adjustments inserted. The agreement between the two smoothed records is now seen to be consistently good, back for many centuries (see *35*

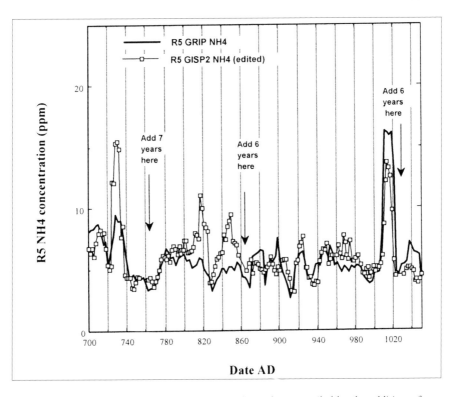

36 How the GRIP and GISP2 ammonium records can be reconciled by the addition of a total of 19 years between the calendar dates 700 and 1050. *Original data obtained from: The Greenland Summit Ice Cores CD-ROM. 1997. Available from the National Snow and Ice Data Center, University of Colorado at Boulder, and the World Data Center-A for Paleoclimatology, National Geophysical Data Center, Boulder, Colorado. Revised dates by this author*

plotted with GISP2 moved back by 19 years). One issue that can immediately be resolved by this move of the GISP2 record is that the lost core section in the sixth century is now seen to span *c.*595–522. Thus the GISP2 record misses both the important 536–45 (proposed comet) event, and the 527+/-1 GRIP volcanic event. Readers should notice that nothing more needs to be done to the GISP2 record to reconcile the two ammonium records back to the fifth century BC.

With the GISP2 record re-dated before AD 1050 we now have a sensible, replicated, ammonium record for almost the whole period back from AD 1640 to around 400 BC.

THE PLAGUE OF THE 660S

Although not illustrated, there is a rise in ammonium in the 660s in both the GRIP core and in the 19-year re-dated GISP2 record. This date is of interest because there is another serious plague recorded in the AD 660s by Bede.[4] It looks as if there is the beginning of a pattern here. Obviously not all ammonium spikes in the ice record are related to plagues. However, it seems that at each of the major plagues ammonium is present. It would be possible to argue that it is really very unlikely indeed to find ammonium at the times of the three pre-defined great plagues of the last two millennia. Also, since we know that there is ammonium in the ice at the time of the Tunguska impact, it can at least *be suggested* that the three plagues may all have been triggered, in some way, by bombardment. (It is impossible to leave the 660s without adding a note with respect to the date. It is suggested that the plague arrived into Ireland on 1 August 664.[5] What are we to make of the fact that the plague is elsewhere called *Lues Inguinaria*, and 1 August is the festival of Lugh?)

THE PLAGUE OF ATHENS

If the reader refers again to *Figures 34* and *35*, it really is pretty obvious that the GISP2 ammonium record is offset from the GRIP record by *about* 19 years; and inserting 19 years into the GISP2 record allows reconciliation between the two cores. So now we know that both the oxygen-isotope and the ammonium records in the two ice cores can be made to fit. So, this must also hold for the sulphate record (and indeed any other chemistry). It had always been assumed that it was volcanoes (i.e. the sulphate from volcanoes) that would form the great link between ice cores. Several seminal papers have been published on this subject by both the American and European groups.[6] Thus, for example, there is that consistent layer of acid in all the ice cores at around AD 1259 (Chapter 13), and we've already seen the issue of the 930s. In fact, moving the GISP2 record, pre-AD 750, back by 19 years makes quite a reasonable job of reconciling the sulphate records as well.

THE SULPHATE AND AMMONIUM RECORDS 1–800 BC

From *Figure 37A* it is evident that the GRIP and 19-year re-dated GISP2 records agree really well back to about 400 BC. Unfortunately, while the GRIP record was replicated by the Dye3 and NGRIP records back to around the start of the present era, before that there is poorer detailed replication. Thus, once we go back into the BC era it is no longer possible to be sure which core is 'correct'. In *Figure 37B* it is evident that the large ammonium spikes in the GRIP and the 19-year re-dated GISP2 records are starting to slip out of phase around 440 BC, 600 BC and 775 BC. This is also consistent with Southon's suggestions. However, as there are no 'fixed points' of any sort this far back in time to act as a check, either record (or both) could have errors. So, it is important to recognise that, even when the 19-year discrepancy is 'fixed', there is still

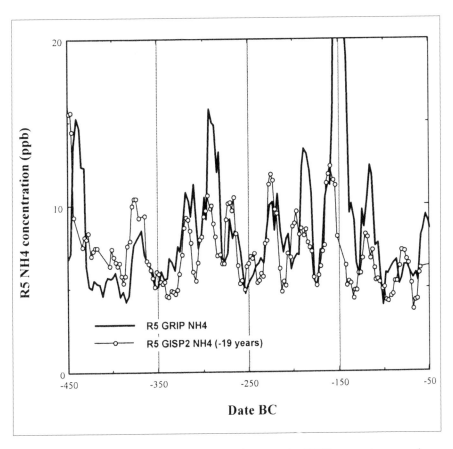

37A The good agreement back to around 400 BC between the GRIP ammonium record and that from GISP2 with the latter shifted back by 19 years. Original data obtained from: The Greenland Summit Ice Cores CD-ROM. 1997. *Available from the National Snow and Ice Data Center, University of Colorado at Boulder, and the World Data Center-A for Paleoclimatology, National Geophysical Data Center, Boulder, Colorado. Revised dates by this author*

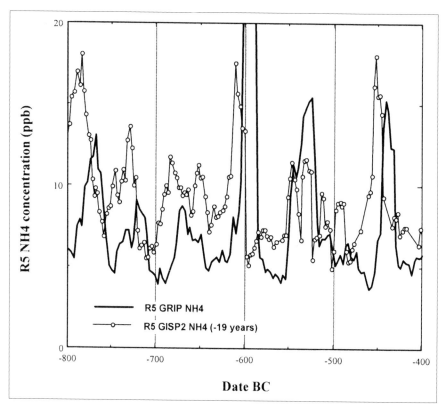

37B Extended data pre-400 BC showing how the two records begin to slip out of phase. With no fixed points available as a check, it is impossible to know whether the problem is in one or both cores

going to be a bit of 'slop' in the ice chronologies (not much, but a bit). When we try lining these records up allowances have to be made within 'a few years'.

Table 6 lists both the sulphate dates and the ammonium dates for the GRIP and the GISP2 cores, for the period 200 BC to 900 BC. In a third pair of columns the GISP2 sulphate and ammonium dates are moved back in time by 19 years. With this done, the dates where the layers make sense between the cores are highlighted in bold. It is very clear that more of the GRIP chemistry dates are duplicated in the 'GISP2 – 19 year' columns and not in the original GISP2 dating. Thus, apart from the visual matching of the ammonium records (*35* and *37*), the agreement between the sulphate records confirms, yet again, that this section of GISP2 core has been misdated by around 19 years.

Now, the reader might ask, 'why am I being dragged through this ice-core chemistry record?' The answer relates to the date 431 BC and it is highlighted in *Table 6* with an asterisk. It seems very likely, given the slight slop in the ice-core dating, that the ammonium at 435 BC in the GRIP core is actually the same layer.

Why would this be important? Its importance would lie in the fact that this 431 BC ammonium date brackets the date of the famous Plague of Athens in 430 BC.

Grip Original		GISP2 Original		GISP2 moved 19 years	
SO4	NH4	SO4	NH4	SO4 (-19)	NH4 (-19)
244		228		247	
	294		279		298
	305				
	314		297		316
	317		299		318
	323		301		320
	374 #		354		373 #
			359		378
421		404		423	
			411		431 *
	435 *		427		446
	438		429		448
	444		431 *		451
			436		455
			440		459
			472		491
			491		510
			496		515
	525				
	528		510		529
	531				
	540		522		541
	543		524		543
	546		527		546
569					
753					
755		736		755	
757		737		757	
888		863		882	

Table 6 Sulphate and ammonium in the GRIP and GISP2 ice-core records (Cols 1-4). Columns 5-6 are the GISP2 record moved back in time by 19 years. Dates in bold suggest better synchronisation at the -19 year position for GISP2 (non-bold dates show less agreement between the datasets). The dates close to 373 BC and 430 BC are highlighted

There is a general acceptance that, whatever the plague was that occurred from 540 onwards, it was broadly a re-run of the Plague of Athens. In fact, some sources *used* to link the plagues of 430 BC, AD 540 and AD 1348 as if they were successive outbreaks of the same disease – bubonic plague. Nowadays it is more usual to highlight the problems in trying to identify what any of the plagues actually were. Here is how Zinsser presents Thucydides' description of the Plague of Athens:

> Early in the summer of 430 BC …. It spread rapidly. Patients were seized suddenly, out of a clear sky. The first symptoms were severe headache and redness of the eyes. These were followed by inflammation of the tongue and pharynx, accompanied by sneezing, hoarseness, and cough. Soon after this … vomiting, diarrhoea, and excessive thirst …. At the height of the fever the body became covered with reddish spots.[7]

This is not dissimilar to the descriptions of the Justinian plague and the Black Death. However it has to be mentioned that recent results on the analysis of tooth pulp, from what appears to be a plague grave in Athens around 430 BC, suggests that these victims succumbed to Typhoid.[8] Irrespective of that possibility, it is true that some people have gone so far as to suggest that the descriptions used in 540 and 1348 were simply re-writings of Thucydides. From our point of view, what has to be most interesting is that *we now have ammonium around the time of four major plagues.* That is *around* 430 BC, in the AD 660s, and specifically *at* 539 and 1348. What are the chances of this occurring unless there is some causal connection?

THE 373–72 BC EARTHQUAKE AND COMET BREAK-UP

In the winter of 373-72 BC a comet was seen at the time of the great earthquake and tidal wave that destroyed the cities of Helice and Bura in Greece (Helice was some 12 stades (i.e. about 2km) from the sea).[9] The Greek writer Ephorus claimed that the comet was seen to split into two parts.[10] So the possibility has to exist, that the earthquake and tidal wave (tsunami) were caused by debris from this splitting comet striking the earth. Obviously we can now look in the ice-core records for ammonium at this date in both the GRIP core and in the 19-year re-dated GISP2 core. Lo and behold, there is ammonium in GRIP at 374.2 BC and ammonium *plus nitrate* in the re-dated GISP2 record at 372.9 BC (*Table 6*; dates highlighted with #). One could be forgiven for thinking that this is more than coincidence. With this ammonium event centred on 373 BC, we seem to have a perfect package:

A splitting comet,

Plus an earthquake,

Plus a tsunami,

Plus both ammonium and nitrate in the ice record.

This looks like a good candidate for one of those 'comet/impact/earthquake/ tsunami' packages that were hypothesised in Chapter 7. Perhaps this actually was another earthquake, apart from 1908, which was not tectonic!

However, before becoming too euphoric it is worth recording one other detail associated with this package. The second-/third-century AD writer Aelian records that five days before the city of Helice was destroyed all the wild creatures from centipedes to martyns 'got on the road and left town'.[11] The problem with this information is that there is every reason to see it as animals detecting pre-earthquake activity, something that has been widely recognised in association with other earthquakes right down to modern times (suggestions are that some animals are sensitive to high-frequency sounds, or some other unusual manifestation, as the pressure on subterranean faults builds up towards slippage). Obviously, if the information about the animals is correct (Aelian was writing about 600 years after the event so there has to be some doubt), then the earthquake simply was an earthquake and not an impact. Equally obviously, it is essential to give all the relevant details. What is not compromised by the animal behaviour is the record of a splitting comet, synchronous with ammonium and nitrate in the Greenland ice. With respect to the splitting of this particular comet, Jonathan Shanklin reports that astronomical opinion has it that one of the fragments became a comet with a roughly 350-year period that returned in the first, fourth, eighth and eleventh centuries, while the other fragment had a period roughly twice as long, and returned in the fourth century and again in 1106 (when it, in turn, broke up).[12] Such observations are relevant because they provide context for any discussions on what did happen in the past.

CONCLUSION

It should by now be clear that there are events involving ammonium and nitrate production that are associated in time with comets and/or earthquakes, e.g. 373-72 BC and AD 1303, where there are no obvious hints of plague. However, we have now seen that there are other events (at AD 1348, in the AD 660s, at AD 540 and around 430 BC) where there is ammonium in the Greenland ice *and* major plague outbreaks. Obviously this needs to be sorted out. Why might some impacts produce 'plagues' while others do not? Irrespective of the answer to this specific question, this has to be a new perspective on the Black Death that was lacking when it was studied only in the isolation provided by looking back from the

present. Recent centuries have failed to adequately enlighten us as to the catastrophic possibilities presented by nature. When the Black Death is seen as simply
another episode in a series of interconnected happenings over many centuries it
begins to make sense. It also becomes clear which parameters need to be studied
if we are to understand it properly. It looks as though the cause was not primarily
a bacterial vector; the bacterial killer may merely have been a symptom; the real
cause may have been something from space.

We could also note again the statement by Thucydides. Why does he say of the
Plague of Athens 'Patients were seized suddenly, out of a clear sky'? We are used
to this form of words in the sense 'it came out of the blue'. How may Thucydides
have meant it? Is it possible that he meant it literally? If he did, then the severe
headaches, the redness of the eyes, the inflammation of the tongue and pharynx,
and the sneezing, hoarseness, and coughing, could have been due to something
in the atmosphere. It only remains to wonder if it really did blow in from a clear
sky.

ROUNDING OUT THE STORY

This chapter will address two issues that contribute to the overall story. One relates to the issue of temperature during the 1340s – was it cold and, if so, why? The other relates to the issue of atmospheric mixing. Atmospheric mixing is a concept bedevilled by prior assumptions. Most people believe that because the wind blows, the constituents of the atmosphere are well mixed. As we shall see, this need not always be the case.

THE TEMPERATURE BUSINESS

The reader is now aware of the previously unknown fact that the first wave of the Black Death sits in a global tree-ring trough, implying a direct environmental component to the story. Tree-ring chronologies from around the world indicate a general decline in ring width on what must have been a fairly massive scale, see *Figures 14* and *15*. This observation, justified in Chapter 2, raises a number of questions. For example, if trees on a large scale are growing less well for several years it is most likely that the global temperature has been turned down. Rainfall has a much more local distribution and it is difficult to see how either more, or less, rainfall could be produced on a global scale. It is also problematic that changes in rainfall would consistently lead to *reduced* growth. So, let's assume that in the later 1340s it got cooler.

There are two main ways of producing cooling. Either the sun provided less warmth, or something was interposed between the sun and the earth's surface – a dust veil of some sort. Can we separate out these two possibilities? This is where the radiocarbon-calibration work and the suggested injection of carbon dioxide into the earth's atmosphere may help. First the carbon dioxide issue. If there really were an injection of 20 billion tons of carbon dioxide into the atmosphere it would pretty certainly have had to come from the oceans. The reason for saying this is that for it to be injected from space it would have required a lump of frozen carbon dioxide approximately 3km in diameter. Allowing that even comet nuclei only have a proportion of carbon dioxide in their makeup, this means that an unrealistically large impact would have to have been involved. Thus we can probably ignore the idea of the carbon dioxide being introduced directly from space.

If we look at the shape of the radiocarbon calibration curve across the 1340s (*16-18*) we see that this is a period where the radiocarbon ages on known-age wood are getting older. Older radiocarbon dates mean that there was less radiocarbon in the wood samples being dated. This implies a dilution of the radiocarbon in the atmosphere by older carbon e.g. carbon dioxide from the oceans which, being older, is already depleted in radiocarbon. There is the additional factor that, normally, less radiocarbon is *produced* when the sun is relatively active, and the strong solar wind is reducing the amount of cosmic radiation reaching the earth's atmosphere to produce the radioactive carbon isotope.

So now we have two issues to play with. The dilution, probably from the oceans and the production, partly related to the activity of the sun. One way to interpret the observed radiocarbon results would be to suggest that the sun may have been *relatively active* at this time. If the sun was *relatively active*, then the reduced growth must have been due to something else; namely, something getting between the sun and the earth's surface. The alternative is the injection of older carbon dioxide from the oceans. Thus either way we look at this, the shape of the radiocarbon calibration curve *tends to support the idea of the earth's atmosphere being loaded with some agent.*

From the point of view of this book, the important observation is the clear ammonium signal spanning 1348 (*Table 5*). So it is reasonable to ask what relationship this ammonium in the atmosphere has with the repetitive, contemporary, descriptions of 'corrupted atmosphere'. Remember the quote:

> This concept of a corrupted atmosphere, visible in the form of mist or smoke, drifting across the world and overwhelming all whom it encountered, was one of the main assumptions on which the physicians of the Middle Ages based their efforts to check the plague.[1]

We now know that there is a physical basis for this belief, and we should not be misled simply because the amount of ammonium in the ice seems relatively small. Depending on the source area of the ammonium, for example if it came from the equatorial region, the signal in Greenland might be lower than was the case with Tunguska simply because the ammonium washes out of the atmosphere pretty rapidly. If the Tunguska ammonium was produced high in the atmosphere (as the nitrate was) then that event took place in an optimum position to allow massive deposition in Greenland. We do not know the source of the 1348 ammonium, unless, of course, we take on board Hecker's statement regarding 'the fiery meteor somewhere in the east'. The problem is that people do not like the idea of corrupted atmosphere because if the agent was in the atmosphere it is automatically assumed that it would have affected everywhere. This as we shall see is not strictly correct.

THE CORRUPTED ATMOSPHERE

How would we get a corrupted atmosphere to kill a lot of people? The most likely mechanism would be through affecting their respiratory system in some catastrophic way. After all, writer after writer on the Black Death makes the point that it is the 'pulmonary' form of the disease that was the dominant killer. This seems to be the 'get out clause' for those who do not like the idea of the disease actually being wind-borne (or, as was said at the time, 'due to poisoned air').

Let's think about this. The disease was for a long time considered to be 'clearly bubonic plague' because there are some descriptions involving buboes. But the disease is spreading too rapidly, and killing too quickly (indeed killing far too high a proportion of its victims) to be classic bubonic plague. So opinion has changed to accommodate these discrepancies. Now it *must* have been the person-to-person variant that was doing the infecting! Here, for example, is what Ziegler says in a few places. When he reads of 65,000 people dying in Marseilles in a month, he says:

> The figure seems improbably high but, as in many sea-ports where bubonic and pulmonary plague raged side by side, mortality was greater than in the inland regions.[2]

Later he says that, as the plague moved north from Paris:

> In this area, exceptionally, the winter checked the violence of the epidemic but with the spring it returned, evidently in its more virulent pulmonary form.[3]

Looking back over those quotations, the reason that pulmonary plague has to be invoked is:

(a) It has to be some form of bubonic plague (in order to sustain the current paradigm), and
(b) It is known that people were dying suddenly and the only easily spreadable form of bubonic plague is the pulmonary or pneumonic form.

And, why has this to be invoked? Because of records such as:

> As late as June 1349 the King authorized the mayor (of Amiens) to open a new cemetery on the grounds that: 'The mortality ... is so marvellously great that people are

dying there suddenly, as quickly as between one evening and the following morning and often quicker than that.'[4]

Here we can see the dilemma for historians locked into a 'bubonic plague' paradigm. The rate of spread – and the speed of death – insists that it would have to be pulmonary bubonic plague. But, the problem with that diagnosis is, with death this fast, there is going to be *no physical evidence* to suggest that the cause was bubonic. Basically, pulmonary plague is being invoked because it has to be, not because of any evidence that it existed. This is an interesting conundrum. Traditionally it was the presence of buboes that suggested the plague was bubonic. Once we move to blaming the bulk of deaths on the pneumonic form, this diagnostic feature disappears from the record. Looked at impartially it seems reasonable to ask: if people were dying from something that was affecting their respiratory system, then why should not the 'something' have been 'corrupted air'? This statement seems reasonable because:

(a) People at the time were pretty adamant that it was 'poisoned air' that was the 'pestilentia'; and
(b) Because there is now a plausible scientific case that extraterrestrial material may have entered the earth's atmosphere at the time, and
(c) Because there is scientific evidence for (at least) ammonium in the atmosphere, specifically at the time of the plague.

At least this is a reasoned argument with some evidence, as opposed to the 'pneumonic plague' dogma. So, just to keep the story simple, how do people react to breathing in ammonia? The answer is, not well. As a gas ammonia will irritate the respiratory tract even at low concentrations. Two thirds of people find a concentration of 50 parts per million (ppm) moderately irritating, while once the concentration reaches around 100 ppm everyone experiences notable irritation of the nose and throat. Higher concentrations, for example above 1500 ppm can cause fluid to accumulate in the lungs and can be fatal through pulmonary edema.[5] It is important to stress the following: it is *not* being claimed here that the Black Death was a mass poisoning by high concentrations of ammonia. What is clear is that there was some ammonia in the atmosphere at the time of the Black Death and it may well be acting as a signpost for other comet-derived chemicals in the atmosphere at the time. However, we still have to work out how this can be related to the historical record of the Black Death and its spread. Only when all the aspects of the story are brought together will we be able to do this.

(Apart from ammonium, it is now known that a range of unpleasant, toxic and evil-smelling chemicals, including hydrogen sulphide and carbon disulphide, have been detected in recent comets. If such chemicals were dumped into the atmosphere by impacts, it might explain frequent references to corrupted or foul atmosphere associated with the Black Death.)

THE GREENHOUSE ISSUE

Referring to *Figures 13-15*, it is very clear that after the global growth-depression of the 1340s there is a general recovery where *all the chronologies show improved growth* in the years from about 1350-5. This was always one of the most surprising things about the tree-ring event across the Black Death. What was it that caused all the chronologies to recover? There have to be two possibilities. The first would be the most outlandish; namely that the growth depression was due to some sort of growth inhibition – poisoning if you like – and that across 1350-5 the 'poison' dispersed. The other alternative is that the trees benefited across 1350-5 from a pulse of 'greenhouse warming'. The reader has to remember that this point of discussion is based purely on the observation of a growth depression in global tree-rings. It is not based on the Black Death having taken place at this time. It is not based on whether or not there is ammonium, or anything else, in the atmosphere at this time. It is purely based on the observed tree-ring downturn and recovery. This is equivalent to posing a question: 'Is it possible that either something poisoned the world's trees in the 1340s, or, that some greenhouse gas was injected into the atmosphere around 1350?'

We now know that there was ammonia in the atmosphere in the later 1340s and that this may only have been a signpost for a pulse of extraterrestrial, cometary, chemistry. We also know that there may well have been pulse of carbon dioxide injected from ocean turnover. If we do not like coincidences, one way to integrate these issues would be to imagine a fragment of comet arriving from space, producing ammonia, injecting unpleasant chemistry into the atmosphere, *and* causing a turnover of the oceans. Note that this scenario does not depend on historical references. It can be derived purely from information from tree-rings and ice cores – there is no human dimension.

RADIOACTIVE ¹⁴C IN THE ATMOSPHERE

One reason why people do not like the idea of the Black Death being due to corrupted atmosphere is the widely held belief that the atmosphere is well mixed. The argument usually goes 'if the plague was in the air, then everyone should have got it; also no-where should have escaped the pandemic'. Here we can add some information hardly known outside the radiocarbon community. When the calibration work (discussed in Chapter 3) was being undertaken, back in the 1970s and 1980s, Pearson and his team used dated Irish oak to measure the past radiocarbon activity. Stuiver, in Seattle, mostly used dated German oak samples, supplied by Bernd Becker. The two sets of results were published in 1986.[6] Although it was found that the overall Pearson and Stuiver calibration curves were essentially identical over thousands of years, there were short periods when the data-sets clearly diverged. *Figure 38* shows such an episode.

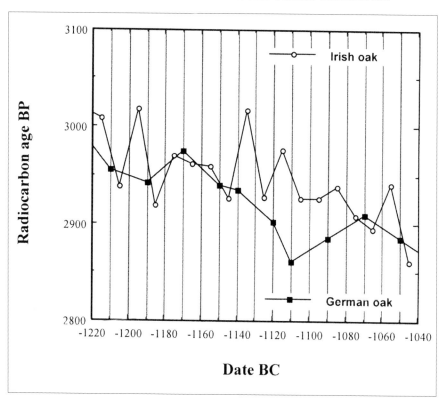

38 Radiocarbon dates on precisely dated Irish and German oak samples show a systematic offset between radiocarbon ages between 1140 BC and 1080 BC implying non-uniform mixing of the atmosphere. *Data from Gordon Pearson and Minze Stuiver*

What is very evident from these radiocarbon measurements on wood of exactly known age is that there is an offset between the results for the Irish and the German wood. For example, from 1140-1080 BC the radiocarbon measurements on German oak samples are older; meaning that there is less radiocarbon in the German samples. Since everything else is constant, the only variable is geographical location. This observation on well-controlled datasets made sense of some other similar findings already in the literature. In fact it gave rise to the first published account of regional radiocarbon offsets.[7]

How do we explain the offset in *Figure 38* if the carbon dioxide containing the radiocarbon is blowing around in the wind? Well, oaks growing in the north of Ireland are subjected to prevailing winds continuously blowing off the Atlantic; for them the atmosphere is indeed 'well mixed'. However, for oaks growing low down in German river valleys, this need not be the case. There they may well be subjected to an atmosphere that included some 'old' carbon dioxide, from rotting humus in valley soils. This old carbon dioxide (involving carbon that is depleted in radiocarbon) would result in older radiocarbon dates for the German samples.

It is clear, therefore, that the atmosphere does not have to be fully mixed; it is quite possible to have areas that avoid mixing (on a bigger scale, it is well known that there is a 'radiocarbon offset' between the two hemispheres presumably brought about by there being more ocean in the southern hemisphere; so there is no special pleading here, offsets are perfectly acceptable scientific observations). This surprising and counter-intuitive finding needs to be stressed. The fact that the atmosphere is not fully mixed, when applied to the 'poisoned air' scenario, allows both the possibility that corrupted air could have affected different areas at different times, and the chance that some areas would be spared.

CONCLUSION

There appear to be reasonable grounds – based on tree-rings, ice cores and radiocarbon – for believing that there was material in the earth's atmosphere, during the 1340s, which contributed to the cooling that seems to have affected the planet. Now, there is evidence to show that having a substance in the atmosphere does not mean that there has to be a uniform distribution of that substance. The radiocarbon-calibration work has shown that it is possible to have trees in different areas 'breathing' atmospheric gases which contain notably different concentrations of the radiocarbon carbon isotope. As shown above, an entire scenario involving tree-ring downturn and subsequent recovery, an injection of carbon dioxide, and the presence of ammonium in the 1348 ice, can be generated without recourse to history.

But, we also know that there are numerous historical references to dust and to 'corrupted atmosphere' associated with 1348. The scientific results indicate that it would be possible to have a 'corrupted atmosphere' that could have affected different areas in different ways – some affected, some spared – and quite possibly in a time-transgressive manner. So, part of the documentary record is highly consistent with the scientific observations. The problem is that the consistency is with the parts of the historical record which are least believed by historians. They are, however, highly consistent with the basic ideas of Hoyle and Wickramasinghe.

As is often the case in research, when a bold theory – such as that proposed by Hoyle and Wickramasinghe – is put forward, it contains several different strands of argument. The problem with bold theories seems to be that if part of the theory is concluded to be wrong, the whole theory is dumped – the baby quite possibly going out with the bathwater. This seems to have been the case with the proposals by Hoyle and Wickramasinghe.[8] They proposed:

(a) That pathogens, including bacteria and viruses, actually occurred in space, in comets, and that these pathogens could rain down onto the earth, and

(b) They also proposed that small particles falling through the atmosphere would tend to descend at different rates in different areas.

When their ideas were looked at by others, it was concluded that the pathogens could not have come from space. For example here is part of what Sagan and Druyan say on the subject:

> There is no report of major epidemics associated – even with a one-year time delay to allow for the bugs drifting down from the stratosphere – with spectacular meteor showers. Moreover, the cometary debris collected by stratospheric aircraft is not reported to contain the charred and mangled bodies of ... pathogens. Scientists examining recovered cometary particles do not seem to be dying of mysterious illnesses. Such facts must be considered among the deficiencies of the hypothesis.[9]

These reasoned arguments seem to put paid to the 'diseases from space' idea. However, we have to note that *they in no way dismiss the secondary proposal* that material entering the upper atmosphere would drift down to the earth's surface at different rates, covering different areas. It is implicit in what Sagan and Druyan say that this part of the hypothesis is quite acceptable. Thus, there is a perfectly viable mechanism available for the selective distribution of poisonous material in both time and space. If that poisonous material was introduced by the insertion of cometary debris into the upper atmosphere, then there is a perfectly viable mechanism available for this selective distribution of *extraterrestrial poisonous material* in both time and space. This is consistent with one major component of the historical record – the 'corrupted atmosphere' references. Moreover, as shown, the historical community seem to have moved to a position where they basically accept that the agent, that was killing people in 1348-9, was transmitted through the air. All in all, the documentary record of the Black Death seems surprisingly consistent with the scientific scenario, viz. *impacts, earthquakes, tsunami and corrupted atmosphere.*

18

TOADS AND SNAKES
AND DRAGONS

There is one last piece of information that is needed to complete the puzzle and it relates to a fundamental issue. When modern readers are presented with a document that mentions toads or scorpions raining down from the sky, they see this as good grounds for dismissing the offending document out of hand. Any ancient writer mentioning rains of frogs is automatically suspect. Until recently this author would have taken the same view. Then, as outlined in this book, the discovery of a core of truth in some dated myths and metaphors raised the spectre that the problem does not lie with the writers of these strange tales. The problem lies with us, and our inability to understand what is being presented to us. This is where the recent work by Barber and Barber is so important, by providing a framework for the understanding of bizarre mythical stories. Readers now know that there is real information in myth and other strange, previously ignored, stories. Things that had been disregarded because they seemed just too bizarre may now, post Barber and Barber, need to be reassessed. The following is a logic chain that may, in the light of some of the information in this book, make some sense. It relates to dragons, but it starts with Roger of Wendover.

In Chapter 6 it was pointed out that Roger of Wendover's history had been summarily dismissed as 'medieval fantasy' by a mainstream British historian. However we now know that Roger's reference to a close comet, blood from the sky and pestilence, in the year 541 appears to be accurate. While leafing through his history (which may indeed be mostly fantasy but certainly survives the 540 test) it was noted that he has another peculiar entry with the date 503. He says:

> In the year of grace 503, a madman in Africa named Olympus, was smitten with a fiery dart from Heaven and consumed, while blaspheming the holy Trinity in the baths.[1]

On its own this seems strange enough to be safely ignored (this author cannot make head nor tail of it). However, it so happens that there is a Chinese story which says:

In the sixth month of the fifth year of the P'u t'ung era [AD 524] dragons fought in the pond of the King of K'uh o (?). They went westward as far as Kien ling ch'ing. In the places they passed all the trees were broken. The divination was the same as in the second year of the T'ien kien era [AD 503], namely that their passing Kien ling and the trees being broken indicated that there would be calamity of war for the dynasty …[2]

It seems that in China in 503 dragons were wrestling in ponds, and where they passed all the trees were broken. The Chinese stories make it clear that 'dragons' are fireballs. A sensible interpretation would be that a bolide burning up in the atmosphere leaves a smoky trail high in the atmosphere. The upper atmosphere winds rapidly turn this dust track into an undulating trail, which appear as a 'dragon'. The dragon proceeds over the horizon (if it explodes closer there are no living eyewitnesses) and results in a fireball. This (or something very like it) is the origin of the 'fire-breathing dragon'. For the observer of this distant impact (remember Tunguska) the ground shakes and lakes seiche (if he or she is close to a body of water). Anyone witnessing dragons crossing the sky *and* a simultaneous seiche in a lake is entitled to describe the happening as 'dragons wrestling in ponds'. The 'trees being broken' also makes perfect sense when it is remembered that the Tunguska fireball flattened 2000sq km of Siberian forest.

So, in China there were fireballs in 503 and now we see that, from somewhere, Roger of Wendover had picked up a story of a man killed by a fiery dart in the same year. Strangely, in Ireland it is recorded that in 503 'Lughaidh (was) killed by lightning at Achadh-farcha, county of Meath.'[3] Given the general paucity of records in the early sixth century, the existence of these three separate stories of things striking from the sky in 503 is remarkable, and again suggests that Roger of Wendover's record is not all fantasy.

This Chinese record alerts us to the fact that in the East dragons, even fire-breathing dragons, can be real descriptions of fireballs from space. The same thing can be found in Russian folk beliefs. For example, one of the first writers on the zoomorphic deities of the Slavs, Afanas'ev (writing in 1852) saw in the folklore:

> … the origins of the dragon from various natural phenomena which seem to con-jure up the image of a flying, fiery beast, scattering sparks: 'The folk imagination … creating mythic images … personified aerial meteors, falling stars and especially lightning … simple folk take falling stars and meteors to be dragons.'[4]

Scholars in the West seem to have lost this knowledge, and now mostly screen dragons – and such like – out of consideration. However, Cantor in his book on *The Black Death and its aftermath* develops an interesting argument in his chapter entitled *Serpents and Cosmic Dust*. He mentions the consensus opinion that the Black Death was bubonic plague spread by rats, but points out that *consensus can be wrong*. Here is a little of what he says:

The earliest medieval explanation for the pestilence was reptiles ....Today the animals associated with the plague are rats and fleas but these did not figure strongly
in the medieval imagination .... Contemporary society looked toward less familiar
beasts dwelling in remote areas that could be identified as the sources or the com-
panions of virulent poisons that had allegedly contaminated the entire atmosphere.
Much emphasis was placed on the sea as the source of infection .... It was also suggested that the reptiles had been released from below ground by earthquakes along
with the corrupt air that caused the disease.[5]

Now in the context of this book, where an *impact/earthquake/tsunami/corrupted
atmosphere* scenario has been developed, it is not hard to see the similarity to
Cantor's points. He is saying that 'serpents from remote areas' (in this case meaning 'dragons from space' which we should understand as 'fireballs from space')
were associated with the poisoning of the atmosphere, with earthquakes, and with
the sea emphatically involved. That is very close indeed to our scenario.

In case the reader thinks that too much is being read into Cantor's 'less familiar
beasts dwelling in remote areas' here is some more about his discussion. Cantor
goes on to say that Louis Sanctus of Beringen (apparently referring to September
1347) mentions rains of frogs, snakes, serpents, lizards and scorpions in the Orient.
What Cantor does at this juncture is interesting. He points out that, in English
bestiaries the 'scorpion' is often illustrated as a kind of 'lizard'. What he is saying is
that all these rains of creatures are actually 'snakes' or 'serpents', i.e. we should not
be misled by the mention of toads or scorpions. But, what he is *really saying* is that
all these 'rains' are of fiery dragons of the type described by the Chinese sources.
So, while references to rains of toads, etc., have caused historians to switch off and
regard such writings as fantasy, in fact all that the medieval recorders were doing
was describing showers of fireballs which caused corruption of the atmosphere.
Interestingly, exactly what Hecker had said.

Such thinking suddenly makes sense of other references. Cantor points to
Gregory of Tours and his story about a great school of water snakes in a Tiber
flood in 589 'and in their midst was a tremendous dragon as big as a tree trunk'.
If, in China, in 503, 'dragons were wrestling in ponds' when in fact 'fireballs were
destroying trees and causing earthquakes and seiches' how then are we to interpret
a story from Rome in 589 when 'schools of water snakes and a dragon were causing a flood' just before a plague? The answer is that modern scholars have to start
getting their heads around the fact that the sky was more active in the past. Impacts
from space, on a variety of scales, were more frequent in the past and *pestilentia*
probably did come from the stars. How chilling to think that the Dominican friar
Bartolomeo may have been factually correct when he wrote that there had been:

> ... massive rains of worms and serpents in parts of China (*Catajo*), which devoured
> large numbers of people. Also in those parts fire rained from Heaven in the form of

snow, which burnt mountains, the land, and men. And from this fire arose a pestilential smoke that killed all who smelt it within twelve hours, as well as those who only saw the poison of that pestilential smoke.[6]

Is this biblical apocalyptic or plain text? On the basis of Cantor's sensible interpretation of how to read such texts, Bartolomeo may have been saying:

> At this time, great showers of fireballs killed many people in parts of China. The accompanying rain of flakes of fire burnt both land and people. Lethal smoke composed of poly-aromatic-hydrocarbons and hydrogen cyanide and ammonia killed anyone exposed to it in a matter of hours.

Could such a thing have happened? Obviously it could have. But all we have to go on is a scientific statement. Here is how a modern astronomer, John Lewis, puts it:

> Yau and his colleagues find three different though mutually consistent records from between the years 1321 and 1368, of a particular fall of iron meteorites that had tragic consequences. One of these reports reads: 'It rained iron to the east of the Erh River. Houses and hill tops were damaged. People and animals who encountered them were mostly killed. It was known as the 'iron rain".[7]

It seems that in the early to mid-fourteenth century things really were falling from the sky.

CONCLUSION

When we start to look at the strange statements from the fourteenth century, they turn out not to be so strange after all. They make reasonable sense when they are looked at in the correct paradigm; that is within the remit of the *impact/earthquake/tsunami/corrupted atmosphere* scenario.

DRAWING TOGETHER THE STRANDS

We now have the ammonium/impact story and it has sufficient support in physical reality to class as a working hypothesis. Science suggests that at the time of the first wave of the Black Death the atmosphere was corrupted. This is consistent with the views of medieval doctors that 'the pestilence had its origin in the air – 'poisoned air' was the widely favoured explanation'.[1] The only question is by what mechanism would this ammonium in the atmosphere have led to widespread mortality? Here a little philosophical musing may be appropriate.

As in any mystery, if the *true answer* could be found it would *explain everything*. If we had the true answer it would explain the weird statements; it would explain the apparent lapses of chronology; it would explain the way the 'plague' spread; it would explain why some areas were spared; it would even explain how the 'plague' could survive in cold northern latitudes. Up until now, there is no single scenario that does this adequately. In fact, the historical approach – looking back from the present, and trying to understand an almost incomprehensible event – seems to be the wrong one. This book has tried to look at the issue from the perspective of the past. When we see that the best records of previous catastrophes are incorporated into myth, metaphor and marginal notes – such as the death of Arthur Pendragon in 539 or 542, or the comment '540; nothing happened worthy of note' – maybe that is how contemporary statements about 1348 also need to be viewed.

As an example of what may be a fourteenth-century metaphor, here is what Konrad of Megenberg (1309-74) wrote about the earthquake of 25 January 1348:

You should also know that the earthquake causes many miraculous things: a vapour coming out from the earth by the earthquake is responsible for transforming human beings and other animals into stone and in particular into pillars of salt. This mostly happens in the mountains, where the people are digging for salt … on some alpine meadows, situated in the higher mountains of Carinthia, about 50 petrified men and cattle had been found. Even milkers would sit beside the cows, both transformed into pillars of salt. Another miracle: due to the earthquake fires may come out of the earth, so that towns and villages will be consumed by it. This fact is caused by the fires inside the earth. A third miracle: during the earthquake sand and dust will come to the surface, so that a whole village becomes absorbed in it.[2]

Such a bizarre idea is ripe to be dismissed out of hand. However, if we were to accept the sixth-century use of metaphor and apply it in this case; is it possible that this description is simply a metaphor for 'Sodom and Gomorrah and fire from heaven'? Could we go further and wonder if Konrad was actually suggesting that the 1348 event was *50 times worse* than the destruction of Sodom? The point being that if we accepted such an idea, even for a moment, it would make some sense of this quotation used by Zeigler:

> In the East hard by Greater India, in a certain province, horrors and unheard of tempests overwhelmed the whole province for the space of three days. On the first day there was a rain of frogs, serpents, lizards, scorpions and many venomous beasts of that sort [*we now know from Chapter 17 to read this as meteors*]. On the second, thunder was heard and lightning and sheets of fire fell upon the earth, mingled with hail stones of marvellous size; which slew almost all from the greatest even to the least. On the third day there fell fire from heaven and stinking smoke, which … burned up all the cities and towns in those parts. (This author's italics.)[3]

Readers not used to this sort of interpretation may find this whole suggestion of metaphor a bit baffling. It is however possible to show that the idea could be on the right lines. The whole story of the destruction of Sodom and Gomorrah is included in chapters 18-19 of the Old Testament *Book of Genesis*. The well-known quotation is:

> Then the Lord rained upon Sodom, and upon Gomorrah, brimstone and fire from the Lord out of heaven. And he overthrew those cities, and all the plain, and all the inhabitants of the cities, and that which was upon the ground. But his wife looked back from behind him, and she became a pillar of salt … and lo, the smoke of the country went up as the smoke of a furnace.[4]

But, apart from the destruction of the cities and their inhabitants by fire from heaven, these two chapters also include the mention of:

A 'herd' of cattle
The term to 'milk'
The number 'Fifty' repeated three times
The term 'Dust and ashes'
The word 'Mountain' repeated three times

How perverse would Konrad of Megenberg have had to be if he was *not* direct-ing us to the message of *Genesis* 18-19? After all, in his completely unbelievable paragraph he includes herd, milking, fifty, mountains and dust and these are the *only* two chapters in the entire bible where these words occur together. As far as this author is concerned, Konrad was telling us in metaphor that the earthquake of 1348 was best described by 'brimstone and fire from the Lord out of heaven'. Now go back to Ziegler's quotation again. There some of the main elements are:

Ziegler   *Genesis*

The slaughter of almost all from the   Destruction of all the inhabitants
greatest to the least

Fire from heaven and stinking smoke   Brimstone and fire from heaven

The burning up of all the cities and towns   Overthrow of the cities

Interpreted in this way, the two sources are so close as to be almost indistinguish-able.

When we couple these descriptions with the ice-core evidence for possible loading of the atmosphere from space across the same period of time, we can start to accept nearly all of Ziegler's accumulated oddities, including the:

floods, earthquakes, subterranean thunder, unheard of tempests, lightning, sheets of fire, hail stones of marvellous size, fire from heaven, stinking smoke, corrupted atmosphere, a vast rain of fire, masses of smoke, heavy mists and clouds, falling stars, blasts of hot wind, a column of fire, a ball of fire, a violent earth tremor, all shortly before the plague arrived.

Given that the new *impact/earthquake/ammonium/corrupted atmosphere* scenario sits comfortably with just about everything in that list, it implies that this scenario is pretty close to the correct answer. If that is the case, then the best clues we had were the comment by Cassiodorus in 537 'But who will not be disturbed … if something mysterious and unusual seems to be coming on us from the stars',[5] and the 1348 definition of the term *pestilència* meaning 'the time of tem-pest caused by light from the stars'.[6] Now, however, we do not need to rely totally on ancient documents when it comes to impacts. As we saw in Chapter 7, recent crater fields are being discovered. We already have Tunguska, Sirente, Chiemgau and Kaali all within the last 3500 years. All of these were over land. As 70 per cent of the earth is covered in water, we can assume that there must have been an absolute minimum of *twelve notable impact events in the last 3500 years*; that is one every 300 years on average! This is an absolute minimum figure because there must be many more crater fields out there, especially outside the developed world.

THE PRACTICALITIES

How would this *impact/earthquake/ammonium/corrupted atmosphere* scenario have worked through the system? The most likely mechanism is that material from impacting comet fragments injected a package of bizarre chemistry into the atmosphere. The recent (4 July 2005) Deep Impact mission to Comet Tempel 1 has shown that comets can contain very large amounts of organic material, including all manner of carbon- and nitrogen-based chemicals (*Appendix 2*). The incoming bolides with their high-energy detonations in the atmosphere can produce ammonium and nitrate to add to the mix. The ozone layer would probably have been affected, just as it was by the nitric oxide generated by the Tunguska fireball in 1908 (as already mentioned, the Tunguska impact probably destroyed around one third of the protective ozone layer).[7] A more intensive disruption of the ozone layer – as could easily have happened in the years 1345-9 (*Table 5*) – may well have subjected humans to unusual levels of ultraviolet radiation, tending to affect their immune systems. Weakened, and exposed to a cocktail of chemicals, in both the atmosphere and, almost inevitably, in their drinking water, they would have been wide open to any disease vector around. One of several diseases, from bubonic plague to anthrax, could have given rise to a percentage of victims with clinical signs of buboes and skin discoloration. Indeed this seems to be the case with later waves of plague. The Great Plague that affected London in 1665-6 seems to have killed at most about 15 per cent of the population of the city (perhaps 65,000 out of 350-400,000).[8]

The key point is that in 1348-9 ordinary diseases may have been killing a percentage of the victims, leaving the infamous clinical signs. Under the cosmic scenario being entertained here the majority of victims in the first wave of the Black Death succumbed to toxic material in the atmosphere, providing an exceptional kill rate. The spread, over a year or so, with its confusing geographical distribution and patchy take-up could easily be explained by material descending from high altitude, as Hoyle and Wickramasinghe had suggested. Moreover, as the regional offsets (demonstrated in the radiocarbon-calibration work) have shown, the atmosphere is not necessarily all that well mixed and it may be possible to have a corrupted atmosphere which is non-uniform, potentially with time-transgressive regional effects. It is probably no coincidence that chronology did become confused in 1348 and 1349 as millions died.

Thanks to Lewis and his inspired suggestion of earthquakes being symptoms of some impacts, it is now possible to envisage packages of information – relating ammonium, nitrates, acid kills, earthquakes and floods (tsunami) – as the signposts for bombardments from space (especially in the absence of any evidence for volcanoes). Now we even have Hughes' changes in the frequency of the recording of comets to tell us that either something fragmented in the inner solar system at around AD 500, and again at around AD 1340+/-40, or, heightened awareness forced people to take more interest in these dangerous objects after those dates.

One other factor which would also make sense is the possible fertilizing effect of all these oxides of nitrogen. The fact that all the global tree-ring chronologies show increased growth just after 1350 (see *13-15*) could well be real evidence for this fertilization. We even have the possibility that a large amount of old carbon dioxide was introduced into the atmosphere at this time (see Chapter 4). Putting all this together, we have across the 1340s first sulphate, then ammonium plus nitrate, then ammonium. We have statements that 1347 and 1348 saw widespread bad harvests with cold and wet conditions. We have the *pestilentia* principally across 1348-9. Then we have a global tree-ring recovery. This picture provides a whole new light on the arrival of Black Death, with a better factual basis than a few infected sailors arriving in three galleys (see below).

Giving credit where it is due, all of this falls so close to the Hoyle and Wickramasinghe idea of 'diseases coming from space', that they must be credited under the rules of 'prior work'. However, although they deserve credit, it is important to make a clear distinction with what is being proposed in this book. They were saying that, in their view, diseases come from space in the form of bacteria and viruses. However, now that we know about the ammonium and acid-kill events associated with a series of major plagues it is perfectly reasonable to argue that people died as a result of something dropping from the sky and corrupting the atmosphere; *just as people in the past had always said.*

THE LIMITATIONS OF THE SCIENTIFIC EVIDENCE

It is widely assumed that everything in the ice cores has been fully analysed. This is not the case. The ice cores have only been analysed for a small suite of possible chemicals. They have not been analysed in any systematic manner looking for things like poly-aromatic-hydrocarbons that are now known to occur in comets. Nor have they been systematically analysed looking for microscopic 'iron' spherules or 'glassy' balls which could well represent an extraterrestrial signal. We know that in the 1960s Chester Langway meticulously melted deep ice from Greenland and reported:

> The most striking particles ... are droplet-globules and spheroidal forms. The morphology of these particles varies ... although perfect spheres are most common .... Microscopic examination also shows that most spherule-globules are opaque and predominantly black or grayish in colour, although dull and vitreous amber, brown, red, and white (transparent and translucent) spherules are present. The lustre of the metallic spherules is usually dull, but black glassy varieties are frequently found .... Almost every black or metallic spherule examined displayed some magnetic susceptibility.[9]

Having undertaken a controlled analysis and looked into the issue of possible contamination, Langway concluded that, in his opinion, the spherules (on average mostly iron and with the vast majority having diameters in the range 5–35 microns) were extraterrestrial in origin. However, it seems that largely because of the fear that the spherules might be modern contamination, Langway's information was never acted upon and no systematic record of these probable extraterrestrial particles has been made. There has to be the real possibility that an incredibly important, continuous, extraterrestrial signal involving everything from a direct rain of comet/asteroidal debris to ablated material from fireballs lies in the stored ice cores. It would be very interesting to know exactly what *is* in the ice at dates such as 540 and 1348.

With the ammonium as a clue, we now have to entertain the possibility that the 'real blood' that fell around 540, the 'smothering cloud of 1014', and the 'reddish air and the dust on the trees' reported in 1348, were actually components of some rain of extraterrestrial chemical soup. In this case the ammonium layers would just be well-dated *signposts*. We even have to entertain the freakish idea that the contemporary references to 'reddish air and dust on the trees' might relate to huge numbers of microscopic particles descending through the atmosphere; a possible addition to the proposed chemical soup.

In Chapter 6 it was noted that McCarthy and Breen now have the sixth-century 'plague' (termed Blefed) arriving in Ireland *at* 540 i.e. synchronous with the outbreak of 'plague' described by Procopius, and essentially synchronous with the large ammonium spike dated to 539 by the ice-core workers. It is not beyond the bounds of possibility that this Irish name for the plague is related to the Old Irish word *bleithid* which relates to a miller or milling. If that were the case, then it might well be that the plague was being likened to a disease normally suffered by millers, i.e. a respiratory disease. In this case also, people may have been breathing a toxic atmosphere, with the ammonium again acting as a signpost. This is where understanding the so-called Black Death of the fourteenth century is helped enormously by looking at it from an earlier perspective. With ammonium and nitrate immediately before the arrival of plague in 1348, and with a definite ammonium signal across the key earthquake date of 25 January 1348, we have every reason to believe that what happened in 1348 was simply a re-run of what had previously happened in and around 540. The implication is that, mixed in with all those spikes of ammonium in the Greenland ice – that were previously thought to be evidence for biomass burning – are a few special events, involving debris from a particular comet source, wherein the atmosphere really was corrupted and people died in huge numbers.

It turns out that the references to 'rains of blood' may not be as outlandish as once thought. In January 2006 two Indian physicists presented a study of the red rains that fell following 25 July 2001 across a few hundred kilometres in India. They observed that the red colorant was *not* Saharan dust, but rather was an estimated 50,000kg of red biogenic 'cells' a few microns in diameter. These cells exhibited a thick outer coat and internal membrane but yielded no evidence for DNA or RNA. It is alleged that the red rain started just a few hours after a meteor airburst on 25 July. The authors propose specifically that this material must have come from a comet and they state that their results support Hoyle and Wickramasinghe's prior ideas![10] Interestingly, this seemingly outlandish suggestion has been taken up by *New Scientist* and treated in a surprisingly open-minded way.[11] Perhaps Roger of Wendover with his 'rain of blood around 540' deserves a more sympathetic hearing than has heretofore been the case.

THE PROPOSAL

At this point, with virtually all the main elements in place, it is necessary to bite the bullet. Frankly, the whole issue of reduced tree growth, impacts, earthquakes and corrupted atmosphere, tied to the earthquake of 25 Jan 1348, founders if we believe the conventional wisdom regarding the contours of the spread of plague, as portrayed by numerous writers. Typical examples are to be found from Carpenter,[12] to National Geographic.[13] All of these show plague emerging from the Black Sea and arriving in Sicily in October 1347; thereafter it spreads to most of Europe. This is the conventional wisdom writ large.

In writing this book it became more and more obvious that a serious look needed to be taken at the dates of the first appearance of the plague. *Figure 39* shows a simplified version of the conventional view of spread. As pointed out previously by Hoyle and Wickramasinghe, some of the contours on such maps do not make a lot of sense. In this conventional view, in later 1347 plague spreads from the Black Sea, *bypassing* Constantinople, and punches out into the Mediterranean to arrive in Sicily. It then spreads in waves which are normally drawn as contours that fail to join up. In *Figure 39* these broken contours are highlighted by question marks. In some ways the map seems to have been drawn to preserve the conventional wisdom rather than in any strictly scientific manner. As luck would have it, Peter Rasmussen attempted to do a more scientific job. In 2000, as part of a BA project, he compiled a list of places with plague start dates and plotted maps month by month from October 1347 right through to 1350.[14] He plotted 'documented outbreaks' as solid black dots and 'possible outbreaks' as diffuse marks. On his October 1347 map his *only* solid 'spots' are on Sicily; the same in November 1347. In December 1347, apart from Sicily he has two solid dots, one at Marseilles and one on the island of Elba. Interestingly, he marks Crete, Constantinople and a few other eastern Mediterranean sites, with only diffuse marks, i.e. unconfirmed suggestions. Here is an independent researcher who has come up with maps that limit the plague, pre-January 1348, to a very tight geographical distribution, essentially Sicily and just possibly Marseilles.

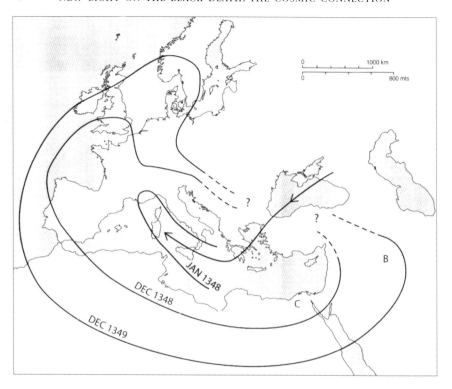

39 A simplified version of the conventional wisdom on the spread of the plague 1347-9 to highlight the anomalous nature of the suggested contours

It is self-evident why and where these dots appear on the 1347 maps. This is the conventional wisdom based on the testimony of the Franciscan Michele da Piazza. He is the one who tells us that in early October 1347:

> Twelve Genoese galleys, fleeing from the divine vengeance which Our Lord had sent upon them for their sins, put into the port of Messina.[15]

Now holding that thought, take a look at *Figure 40*. In this figure it is assumed, on the basis of the comet/ammonium/earthquake scenario developed in this book that the main element of the plague was corrupted air, and it arrived through loading of the atmosphere in January 1348. The figure ignores Rasmussen's late 1347 dates for Sicily but includes his wide spread of dots for places affected in the month of January 1348 (Cyprus has been added, based on the quotations in Chapter 8). The normal contours for the spread of plague up to December 1348 and 1349 are also presented. The big difference is that in this figure, with no 1347 component, the contours make sense and can be drawn as continuous lines.

This means that essentially the only thing standing in the way of the plague actually having arrived in January 1348 is Sicily. Note that if we were to take Sicily out of the equation, the whole chain of Black Sea – Genoese galleys – plague ridden sailors – plague-bearing rats would collapse. Then it would be quite plausible that the plague that affected Europe was a direct consequence of something triggered by the earthquake (impact?) of January 1348. As indeed the author of a German treatise said at the time:

> I say it was the vapour and corrupted air which has been vented – or so to speak purged – in the earthquake that occurred on St Paul's day, 1348.[16]

This line of thinking forces us to have a fresh look at the details of Michele da Piazza's information about the plague in Sicily. Was da Piazza reliable? He paints a graphic picture of the awfulness faced by the Messinese. People were dying in large numbers, so the survivors left the city and spread across the island. If that was the total of his testimony there would be few grounds to question his reliability. However, da Piazza then enters into a long story of how the people of Messina decided that if they could borrow the statue of the virgin Agatha from Catania 'the city (Messina) will be saved completely from this disease'. This is a strange thing to say when he has already stated that Messina had been abandoned because of the 'enormous mortality'. He then goes on to lose any credibility because he says this:

> Several of the Messinese in Catania addressed pious requests to the Patriarch … that he would personally carry the relics of the virgin Agatha to Messina…The Patriarch … agreed ….The holy virgin Agatha, aware of the deep seated deceit and cunning of the Messinese, directed her prayers to God, who arranged it that the whole body of citizens … wrested the keys from the keeper of the church, they roundly abused the Patriarch, declaring that they would see him dead before they let the relics go to Messina.[17]

How does a modern researcher treat the validity of a writer who believes that he can *know the thoughts of*, and indeed *speak for*, a long-dead saint? I suspect we can dismiss him out of hand, especially when he goes on to tell us:

> The Patriarch duly arrived in Messina with the holy water and cured all sorts of sick people in great numbers by sprinkling them with holy water and making the sign of the cross.[18]

This does not agree with his previous assertion that most people had left the city because of the huge death toll. Nor is it sensible to assert that the plague could be cured in this simplistic way. In the end da Piazza's text – with more responsive statues, and even demon dogs with swords – becomes so bizarre that there is no point in this author bothering to write it out (there are three full pages sprinkled

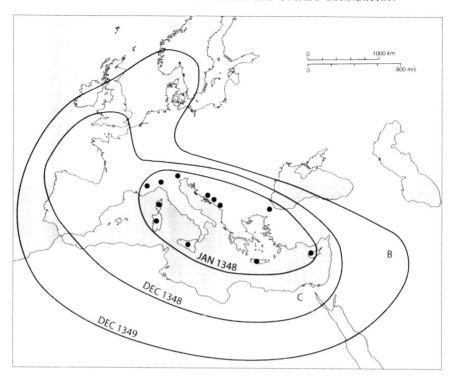

40 Suggested consistent contours of the spread of the plague assuming the true start was in January 1348, not late 1347. This would be consistent with a pathogen descending through the atmosphere as first suggested by Fred Hoyle and Chandra Wickramasinghe. The black dots are mostly from Peter Rasmussen's list of definite first occurrences

with nonsense). He was, after all, writing about 10 years after the events he is allegedly describing. However, da Piazza does tell us that Duke Giovanni, who had hidden in the wild in an attempt to avoid the plague, finally died of it and was buried in April 1348. By doing this he moves the only factual item in his discussion away from 1347 and into the spring of 1348.

Given all that, and on the basis that the main source of information for the arrival of plague in October 1347 was Michele da Piazza, it would be unsafe to believe that plague was in Sicily as early as October 1347. After all, the conventional October 1347 wisdom (*39*) forces us to believe that the plague crossed the Black Sea and travelled to Sicily without infecting Constantinople or anywhere else on the way. It then had to rapidly re-flux throughout the Mediterranean, including Constantinople. This is where Ziegler's tone about infected galleys seems particularly relevant:

It is not necessary to believe, with the Chronicler of Este, that these ill-fated galleys, with the crews dying at their oars, somehow contrived to spread the plague to 'Constantinople, Messina, Sicily, Sardinia, Genoa, Marseilles and many other places'.[19]

Indeed the new January 1348 scenario it is entirely consistent with Ziegler's direct statement:

> By the spring of 1348 the Black Death had taken a firm grasp in Sicily and on the mainland.[20]

It would appear that Deaux found the same thing, because he states clearly that:

> Although one report says that the first deaths were as early as November 1347, it is generally agreed that the plague was not established in Marseilles until January of the next year.[21]

It seems that there is no good evidence, *at any time before January 1348*, for the plague that swept across Europe in 1348-9. Moreover, it was in January 1348 that a widely felt earthquake, when coupled with the occurrence of ammonium in Greenland ice, offers the possibility that the *pestilentia* that did arrive was something borne in the air due to the impact of a fragment (or fragments) of a comet.

In case anyone missed that last point. The plague that ravaged Europe in 1348 and 1349 *was probably not bubonic plague* (because it no longer needs to be). Similarly, it did not need to come from Asia by the normally suggested route, because that route is probably a *post facto* reconstruction to fit the conventional 'bubonic plague' wisdom. All of that may well need to be set aside. What we do need is proper, total, analysis of the ice cores to find out just what was in the atmosphere at AD 1348, 1014, 626, 539 and 430 BC.

CONCLUSION

The original idea in writing this book was that it would be possible to catalogue a range of environmental events in *the run-up to* the 1340s, and these would set the scene for the arrival of the plague. As it has turned out, the logic of this story is that there does not need to be any run-up to these plagues. They simply arrive 'out of the blue' probably delivered by cometary agents exactly consistent with Gibbon's statement:

> I shall conclude this chapter with the comets, the earthquakes, and the plague, which astonished or afflicted the age of Justinian.[22]

'Comets, earthquakes and the plague' – how did he get it so right, even down to the right order? Or again there is Hecker's (normally ignored like Gibbon's):

fiery meteor, which descended on the earth far in the East … [and] … destroyed
everything within a circumference of more than a hundred leagues, infecting the air
far and wide.

'Fiery meteor, destruction, and infected air' – where did he get this information
from? Interestingly, Deaux more or less got it right on his first page:

The first records came out of the east … descriptions of the storms and earthquakes,
of meteors and comets trailing noxious gases that killed trees and destroyed the
fertility of the land.[23]

We can now see how this basic message was repeated again and again; so often
in fact that it borderlines on the bizarre that historians could not see there might
be a core of truth. For a final example here is a statement from Lynn Thorndike,
writing in 1934. She cites a late fifteenth-century abbot, Trithemius, reiterating
information from Giovanni Villani who died in 1348:

Trithemius further states, as Villani had at the time, that in 1347 a vast vapour from
the north settled over the earth to the great terror of those who saw it, and that
some writers mention that in this year innumerable minute forms of animal life
(*quasdam minutas bestiolas*) fell from heaven to earth in the orient and produced the
pest by their corruption.[24]

Given that the use of the year '1347' could encompass a period up to March 1348,
this seems entirely consistent with Gibbon, Hecker, Deaux and Ziegler. Were
Hoyle and Wickramasinghe correct? Of course they were, almost. The correct
answer was '*comets, meteors, earthquakes, tsunami and noxious gases, with just the possibility of some biotic material from space*'. It is important to remember that these key
issues were not deduced from the historical record. They were deduced from the
tree-ring downturn and from the analysis of ancient carbon dioxide, and ammonium, in the ice caps; from the radiocarbon-calibration curve, and from some
largely theoretical considerations regarding whether all earthquakes are solely
tectonic in nature, i.e. the key issues have been deduced from a variety of *scientific*
endeavours. Yet we know from the historical record that in January 1348 there
was a major earthquake just as the 'plague' was starting. We know that at least one
person at the time thought that the plague was a direct result of the earthquake.
We know that someone at the time thought that a black comet was involved.
There even appear to be records of a fiery meteor at the time that caused the air
to be infected. Thus one possible interpretation of the *historical record* would be
that the Black Death somehow involved comet or meteor impacts, earthquakes,
and corruption of the atmosphere. Historians have felt obliged to mention all of
these factors but clearly have not believed that they could actually be true. We

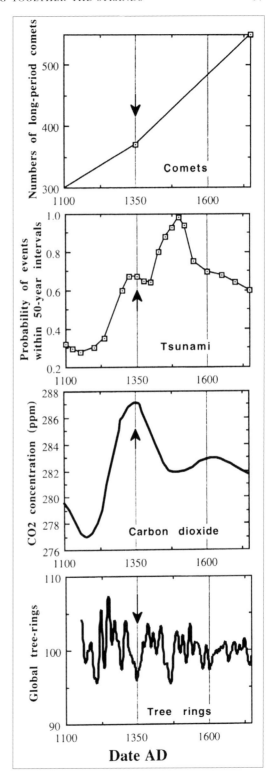

41 Figures 18, 23 and 32 plotted with the smoothed mean global tree-ring curve from Figure 15, showing how independent scientists have introduced suggestions of a global environmental downturn, comet frequency change, tsunami probability, and carbon dioxide enrichment (consistent with an ocean turnover event) at around AD 1350

now know, courtesy of the tree-rings and the ice cores that the ancient writers were probably doing their best to give us an accurate report on what happened.

FINALLY

If we review the significant aspects of the Black Death story that have emerged in this book, any solution to the conundrum of the Black Death now has to take account of the following in the mid-fourteenth century:

> There was a global tree-ring downturn followed by a universal recovery
>
> There were references to things falling from the sky
>
> There were references to a corrupted atmosphere
>
> There was an actual Comet Negra in 1347
>
> There was a change in the frequency of long-period comet observations
>
> There was a major earthquake on 25 January 1348
>
> There was a sub-peak in tsunami occurrence
>
> There was an increase in CO_2 suggestive of ocean turnover
>
> There was ammonia in the atmosphere across 1348
>
> There was a pestilence interpreted by modern historians as pneumonic, i.e. mostly air-borne
>
> There is now a serious suggestion that biogenic organisms can enter the earth's atmosphere from space

That this list is reasonable is reinforced by lining up several previous figures, as in *Figure 41*. In this compilation we see that *totally independent workers* studying comets, tsunami, carbon dioxide and tree rings all observe something happening around the time that the Black Death decimated human populations. Virtually the only thing standing in the way of the *pestilentia* being the direct result of an impact on 25 January 1348 is the dubious testimony of Michele da Piazza.

It seems inescapable that the history of the fourteenth century (and quite a number of other centuries) must now begin to take account of the records that are written in both the trees and in the ice. It really does appear that the key issues, previously missing in considerations of the Black Death, are *comets, impacts, earthquakes, and corruption of the atmosphere.*

The amusing thing about such a conclusion is that Thomas Short, the 'discredited' eighteenth-century compiler of historical information, came very close to discovering this two and a half centuries ago; he just did not know how to interrogate his own data properly, see *Appendix 4*.

POSTSCRIPT

It is increasingly evident that intellectually the world is divided into two. There are those who study the past, in the fields of history and archaeology, and see no evidence for any human populations ever having been affected by impacts from space. In diametric opposition to this stance there are those who study the objects that come close to, and sometimes collide with, this planet. Some serious members of this latter group have no doubt whatsoever that there must have been numerous devastating impacts in the last five millennia; the period of human civilization. In a paper published in 2005, David Asher and colleagues have looked at the objects that are known to have come close to the earth in recent times.[1] They conclude, based on various strands of evidence (for example, the number of meteorites discovered on earth that originated on the moon) that the average time between impacts on earth is no more than 300 years, probably less. Their conclusion is remarkably similar to the 'off the cuff' estimate given in Chapter 19 that was based on different criteria.

These estimates of the frequency of impacts sit very comfortably with the comet/ammonium story developed in this book. Here is another example of why that story might be on the right lines. It so happens that in 2004 astronomer Peter Jenniskens published a paper wherein he proposed that the Quadrantid meteor shower (which normally peaks on 3 January each year) originated from a small body, a minor planet, named 2003 EH. This object, which was discovered in 2003, was in a high-inclination, comet-like orbit that fits with the orbit of the Quadrantids. By projecting the orbits back in time, Jenniskens found that:

> … we cannot exclude that (comet) C/1490 YI was a prior sighting of the Quadrantid parent at the epoch when it created the shower.[2]

This is science speak for 'the Quadrantid meteor shower was created when the comet C/1490 YI broke up early in 1491'. The 'epoch when it created the shower' simply means that the comet broke up in some way, shedding debris. Comets are named for the year in which they were first observed and this is how it was recorded in 1490:

> ... a bright comet [was] observed from China, Korea and Japan between Dec 31.5, 1490 and Feb. 12.5, 1491 [and] passed perihelion on January 08, 1491.[3]

Referring to the American GISP B ice-core chemistry record[4] we find that at a depth of 458.1–459.6m there is *both* elevated ammonium and nitrate. This layer dates between 1490.4 and 1491.9 (centre date 1491.15). Indeed these are the highest ammonium values between 1429 and 1536 and the highest nitrate values between 1427 and 1617. Moreover, as if that is not enough, Schaaf lists the closest *known* approach of a comet as that of comet 1491 II which passed within a mere 1.4 million kilometres of earth on 20 February 1491.[5] It looks as though we get two chances for a comet to have delivered ammonium to the atmosphere in 1491. In this case there is even a sharp growth downturn in European oak at the same time, see *Figure 42*.

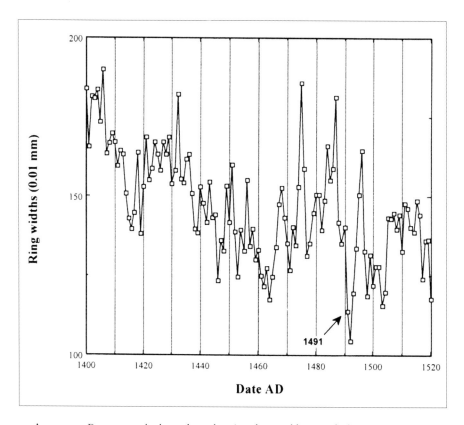

42 An average European oak chronology showing the notable growth downturn in AD 1491

So, again, as we saw with respect to 373-2 BC (Chapter 16), when a comet is found to have broken up – giving rise to a well-known meteor shower – we find that there is both ammonium and nitrate in an ice-core record at the same time.

There really is enough information about comets, earthquakes and ammonium to permit the quite serious suggestion that the Black Death was due to an impact by comet debris on 25 January 1348, as witnessed by the major earthquake on that day. Critics will dismiss this scenario by saying that there were no reports of an impact associated with the earthquake. This is where the Sodom and Gomorrah 'metaphor' of Konrad of Megenberg, used in direct reference to the 25 January earthquake, may be significant (see Chapter 19). 'Sodom and Gomorrah' means 'brimstone and fire out of heaven'. The date is exactly right.

APPENDICES

APPENDIX I

The issue of diseases from space
The principal champions of this idea were Sir Fred Hoyle and Chandra Wickramasinghe. The easiest way to understand the debate is to note that a lot of astronomers, and others, now believe that comets supplied the water and organic materials onto the surface of the early earth that allowed life to develop. This is because from its formation, about 4.5 billion years ago, down to around 3.8 billion years ago the earth was effectively kept molten. So no water could exist on the surface. After major bombardment stopped (as most of the debris left over from the formation of the solar system was finally mopped up by the orbiting planets) the surface cooled. Almost immediately oceans existed. The only way this could have happened was if the water was provided by comets colliding with the cooled early earth. As can be seen from *Appendix 2*, comets contain large reservoirs of organic material. So, rather than thinking that life was triggered in some inorganic soup on the early earth, it is now widely considered that the organic soup was also provided by comet impacts. This makes it much more understandable that, as geologists have observed, as soon as the planet cooled the first signs of life appeared virtually immediately. Hoyle and Wickramasinghe were quite content with this idea. However it is fair to say that they considered things to be just a little more extreme. In their view life could have evolved in the warm interiors of large comets and could have arrived in the form of bacteria and viruses. So, in recent decades it has become acceptable to at least contemplate whether life might exist quite widely in space. This idea is termed pan-spermia (i.e. life is widespread in the universe albeit mostly at a primitive level as in bacteria and viruses).

However, as pointed out in Chapter 16, the idea of diseases from space is largely discounted by mainstream scientists. This, of course, does not mean that, from time to time, all manner of chemicals that might be detrimental to human life cannot rain down from space as fragments of comets enter the earth's atmosphere. Not only can they rain down, apparently they have rained down on a number of occasions most notably around AD 540 and in 1348.

APPENDIX 2

Some recent findings about a comet
After five years of preparation NASA launched its 'Deep Impact' mission to Comet Tempel 1 on 12 January 2005. The spacecraft was set to meet up with the nucleus of the

comet six months later as the comet passed on one of its 5.5-year passages around the sun. As the craft approached the comet at 25km per second (the comet is travelling at 35km per second, so the impact is actually the comet hitting the spacecraft at a velocity of around 10km per second – a high-energy impact by any standards; for comparison a high speed head-on car crash would take place at about 0.07 km per second) it separated into two sections, an impactor and an observer. On 4 July 2005 the comet and the impactor collided, with the impactor craft taking pictures as it approached the comet nucleus and the other craft observing and analysing. The whole operation worked like clockwork.

The nucleus of Tempel 1 is irregularly shaped and has a volume of almost exactly 3 cubic kilometres. It is extremely dark and exhibits a range of craters and smooth planes. When the spacecraft impacted it threw out a first pulse of around 10 tons of hot ejecta (the result of the impact) followed by around 10,000 tons of cold ejecta. The surprise was that everything that came out was in the form of dust a few microns (millionths of a metre) in diameter. What was learned? Although the analysis of the data from the encounter will take years, initial findings are profoundly important. The nucleus is about 75 per cent empty space. The particles that make it up are held together only by weak gravity. But, frighteningly, preliminary analysis shows that the comet is made up of around 25 per cent water-ice, and around 75 per cent organics and silicates. The preliminary list of organics includes carbon-based forms, such as C_2H_2, HCN, CH_3CN, as well as carbon dioxide and sulphur dioxide.[1] The NASA Website elaborates further with a list including clay particles, iron-containing compounds, carbonates, crystallized silicates and polycyclic hydrocarbons.[2] Altogether not a package that anyone would want dumped into the earth's atmosphere.

In many ways the Deep Impact results were not all that much of a surprise. Lifting a 1953 book entitled *The Comets and their Origins*, it transpires that 50 years ago it was already being stated:

> The accepted view of the nature of comets is that they are loose swarms of separate particles, probably of very different sizes, separated by distances great in comparison to their own diameters and accompanied by more or less dust and gas …[3]

Similarly it was known from studies of emission spectra that the general shape of the chemistry of comets could be summed up as:

> … involving mainly carbon, hydrogen, nitrogen and oxygen, and the presence of such molecules as CH, CH+, CH_2, CN, C_2, NH, NH_2, OH and OH+ … NH molecules can only result from photo-dissociation of chemically stable molecules liberated from solid constituents of the comet.[4]

All of this sounds very consistent with the 75 per cent empty space, the micron-sized dust and the organic compounds now observed in Tempel 1. Overall, there seem good grounds for imagining that ammonia (NH_3) or ammonium (NH_4) is present in comets in some quantities, and the observed NH compounds may be dissociating from solid ammonium.

APPENDIX 3

Daniel Defoe's journal relating to the Great Plague of 1665 was published in 1722. His status as an eyewitness is stated on the title page 'A Journal of the Plague Year ….

Written by a citizen who continued all the while in London.' The Journal connects us to the issue of the Black Death because it was written by someone who had survived what is normally taken to be the last significant outbreak of the 1348 pandemic. There are a couple of passages that seem relevant to the current book, and they are quoted here as Defoe wrote them. They give a flavour of the human response to unaccountable phenomena which can have changed little in the three centuries following the start of the Black Death. However, there is no doubt that the comets mentioned did exist and recent research has indicated that it is possible under some circumstances to 'hear' a comet.[1]

Defoe on forerunners of the Plague

But I must go back again to the beginning of this surprising time: while the fears of the people were young, they were increased strangely by several odd accidents, which, put together, it was really a wonder the whole body of the people did not rise as one man, and abandon their dwellings, leaving the place as a space of ground designed by Heaven for an *Akeldama* (a 'place of blood' or a 'cursed place'), doomed to be destroyed from the face of the earth; and all that would be found in it would perish with it ….

In the first place, a blazing Star, or Comet, appeared for several months before the Plague, as there did the year after another, a little before the [Great] Fire. The old women, and the phlegmatic hypochondriac part of the other sex, whom I could almost call old women too, regarded (especially afterward, though not till both those Judgments were over,) that these two Comets passed directly over the City, and that so very near the houses, that it was plain they imported something peculiar to the City alone: that the Comet before the Pestilence was of a faint, dull, languid colour, and its motion very heavy, solemn, and slow; but that the Comet before the Fire was bright and sparkling, or, as others said, flaming, and its motion swift and furious; and that, accordingly, one foretold a heavy Judgment, slow but severe, terrible, and frightful, as was the Plague; but the other foretold a stroke, sudden, swift, and fiery, as the Conflagration was; nay, so particular some people were, that as they looked upon that Comet preceding the Fire, they fancied that they not only saw it pass swiftly and fiercely, and could perceive the motion with their eye, but even [that] they heard it; that it made a rushing mighty noise, fierce, and terrible, though at a distance, but just perceivable.

I saw both these Stars, and I must confess, had so much of the common notion of such things in my head, that I was apt to look upon them as the forerunners and warnings of God's judgments; and especially when after the Plague had followed the first, I yet saw another of the like kind, I could not but say, God has not yet sufficiently scourged the City.

Defoe on the abating of the Plague

In the middle of their distress, when the condition of the City of London was so truly calamitous, just then it pleased God, as it were by his immediate Hand, to disarm this enemy; the poison was taken out of the sting: it was wonderful! Even the Physicians themselves were surprised at it: wherever they visited, they found their patients better, either they had sweated kindly, or the tumours were broke, or the carbuncles went down, and the inflammations round them changed colour, or the fever was gone, or the violent head-ache was assuaged, or some good symptom was in the case; so that in a few days, every body was recovering; whole families that were infected and down, that had ministers praying with them, and expected death every hour, were revived and healed, and none died at all out of them.

Nor was this by any new Medicine found out, or new method of Cure discovered, or by any experience in the operation, which the Physicians or Surgeons attained to; but it was evidently from the secret invisible Hand of Him, that had at first sent this disease as a Judgment upon us.

APPENDIX 4

Thomas Short's *A General Chronological History of the Air, Weather, Seasons, Meteors, Etc.* was published in 1749. Ostensibly this is a listing of notable events from the time of the Flood in 2349 BC through to AD 1748, with particular emphasis on the great plagues of history. As noted in the text, Short had been classed as unreliable by Britton, and his history is generally regarded as unreliable. Unreliable in the sense that he does not give sources for many of his entries, which have in consequence proven un-checkable. However, from our point of view, what is most interesting about Short's book is that after listing all the happenings in history he settles down, on page 323 of Volume II, to set down some *General Observations and Inferences from the History of the Air and its Effects.* This is a chapter in which Short looks at his assembled phenomena and dates to see if there is any hint of cause and effect. In a sense he was testing the paradigm that disease was due to some 'corruption of the atmosphere'. It is interesting to see how he got on.

He starts by pointing out that hot or wet seasons can cause disease, though this is at a low and local level. He then moves on to (page 331-2) how 'Several Epidemics have undeniably arisen from other causes than the Air'. He provides a long list of things that can promote disease of which a few are:

> Trade, Navy, Strangers … putrified Carcases of Animals … great Inundations in marshy, flat Countries, very high Tides that throw Multitudes of Fish ashore in hot Weather … Locusts, or other Insects … dying on Heaps and putrifying … opening long shut-up vaults; or from Earthquakes or Chasms in the earth

He then gives various examples. It is clear that this is not what he really wants to deal with. In his section 67 (page 345) he makes his intention clear.

> In our Quest of natural Causes, we shall run over the most considerable Meteors and the Phenomena in the Table (his compilation), and see which of them do most ordinarily produce Epidemics and Mortality; and whether they produce them alone, or attended by other Concomitants; and we think it cannot be denied, that what Meteors, Seasons, or Changes of Air, may produce Diseases alone, may be allowed to do the same when conjoined to other Circumstances; on the contrary, such Things as do not ordinarily, or very rarely occasion Epidemics when alone, cannot justly be charged with them, when accompanied with such circumstances, that often produce Diseases.

In other words he wants to try to deduce the important causes of Epidemics, and he makes it clear that he wants to adopt a scientific approach:

> Now what these Things are that generally give Rise to such common Calamities, shall be fairly and faithfully tried from History and Facts alone. By comparing the preceding Tables of Earthquakes and Epidemics together, we shall find that though several of them have happened in the same Year, yet few of them fell both in the same country; but still fewer where the Earthquake was neither preceded nor attended by such Things as are mostly the Forerunners of a great Mortality; but fewest of all where the last immediately succeeded the other.

That is, having compiled his Tables of phenomena, and their dates, he can now interrogate the accumulated data searching for patterns that might suggest cause and effect based purely on the facts of history. Clearly, from what he states about earthquakes he could not find any reasonable case to blame earthquakes for consistently happening just before epidemics. He spends more than four pages giving examples of earthquakes that *followed* epidemics, and hence could not have caused them, e.g 'the Fevers which began in *England* in *May 1727* (could not have been caused by) that Earthquake in *Warwickshire, July 17* (1727)'. So Short, with a few exceptions, ruled out earthquakes as a common cause of epidemics. In fact, he states that out of 500 or 600 earthquakes 'not above 15 or 16 of them alone have preceded immediately before Epidemics'. He then goes on to rule out astrological conjunctions, seasons, comets, northern lights and fiery meteors. Though he does say:

> From about 104 Instances in the table of fiery Meteors, I cannot discover them to be any Forerunners or Presages of general or particular Calamities to Nations or People, whatever Indication they may be hereafter of the general Conflagration. Of 78 notable Conflagrations of the Heavens, though they coincided with several epidemical Years, yet most of the Epidemics were either begun or over before the Conflagrations happened, as in 1347, 1574, 1623, 25, 26, 1737, etc.

Next he rules out unnatural colours of the Sun and Moon, burning clouds, falling stars, thunder and lightening. Then, having tabulated the 431 epidemical years in his record and recorded the most common coincident factors he concludes:

> Therefore from these Evidences, that the common and ordinary natural Causes of Epidemics are from Experience and Fact found to be long and great Rains, Droughts, and Heat, Frosts and their Consequences, Famines, Locusts tempestuous and unequal Seasons, and Communication from other Parts.

Readers of this present book could take from Short that there is no good case for linking comets, or meteors, or conflagrations of the heavens to epidemics. However, it is clear from Short's work that all of this deduction is *in general*. Note how he does mention that *the epidemic of 1347 had already begun before the conflagration happened*. If the idea suggested in this book were taken at face value, the great killer of 1348 and 1349 may not have begun before Short's 'Conflagration of Heaven' of 1347. This is a case where the precise chronology of events has to be critical. Thus, this would seem to be a good place to look again at Short's compilation, but in a different way. He looked at *all* the cases of epidemics when compiling his 'statistics'. What happens if we look only at the two great universal plagues, i.e. those of 540 and 1348-50?

Short's compilations immediately before the great plagues are:

> 540 - 'A great Comet appeared. Fiery Battles, with abundance of Blood, were seen in the Air'.
> 1347 - 'In *England*, the Year that it came hither, (*viz. September* 28, 1347) it rained from *Christmas* till *Midsummer*, without one fair Day, hence great Floods. In *France*, besides the Rains, in *August* was seen the terrible Comet called *Negra*. In December appeared over Avignon for the Space of an Hour, a Pillar of Fire, the Sun being up. There were many and great Earthquakes, Tempests, Thunders and Lightnings ... some Chasms in the earth sent forth Blood ... Terrible Showers of Hail ... in Germany it rained Blood; in France Blood gushed out of the Graves of the Dead, and stained the Rivers crimson: Comets, Meteors, Fire-beams, Corruscations in the Air, Mock-suns, the Heavens on Fire'

Thus, if Short had asked himself what had taken place just around the time of the start of the two great universal plagues, rather than looking at all the cases of epidemics, he might have recognised, from his own compilation, that these outstanding plagues could have had an extraterrestrial cause.

The Plague of Athens

In his compilation Short devoted a lot of space to the plague of 430 BC, i.e. the other plague that is often cited as being in the same league as the two great plagues of the current era. He says something quite interesting:

> *Thucydides* tells us, that in the 5th Year of the *Peloponesian War*, there were several Shakings of the earth, and the plague that had not been quite extinguished broke out again at that time, and continued about a Year, which being the 33rd Year of *Hippocrates's* Age, and the Year of the Earthquake and Comet mentioned by him, as well as his malignant Year, when he was at *Thasus* … But the Comet and Earthquake that *Aristotle* says happened in Winter, was in the 87th Year of *Hippocrates's* Life, and the 370th or 373rd before *Christ*.

Short was touching on an issue which apparently still exercises scholars today, namely, what did *Thucydides* owe to *Hippocrates*. But, of course, what is interesting is the accuracy of Short on the one hand, and the fact that he had noted another 'Comet and Earthquake' reference in the vicinity of the Plague of Athens on the other. If he had looked only at the 430 BC, AD 540 and AD 1348 plagues he might well have recognised the common components.

APPENDIX 5

This is for those who like coincidences. After the text of this book was completed in early March 2006 the author was in the Oxfam Bookshop in Belfast. An antique leather binding stood out on the religious shelves. The book was priced at 50p, presumably because the front board was missing. It was an 1814 English translation of a German work, originally published in Hamburg in 1784, entitled: *Reflections on the Works of God in Nature and providence, for Every Day of the Year*. The author Christopher Sturm had produced 366 short expositions for the days of the year, each on the theme of some wonder of creation. Opposite page 75 was a picture of a comet linked to a three-page piece on the same subject.

The day chosen by Sturm for his exposition *Of Comets* was January XXV. If this was a random choice then the odds on him picking that date have to be 366 to 1. There is, of course, an alternative explanation: perhaps Sturm knew something about St Paul's Day, 25 January, involving a comet. In his exposition he shows a surprisingly modern understanding of comets and also reminds us:

> Many consider a Comet, as the forerunner of heaven's judgments. Some read in it the destiny of nations, and the fall of empires. To others, it is a presage of wars, plagues, inundations; in a word, of the most formidable scourges.

Coincidence? Maybe, or then again, maybe not.

ENDNOTES

INTRODUCTION

1   Hecker, J.F.C. 1834 *The Black Death in the Fourteenth Century* (trans. Babington, B.G.). Sherwood, Gilbert and Piper, London
2   Arrizabalaga, J. 1994 Facing the Black Death: perceptions and reactions of university medical practitioners. In *Practical Medicine from Salerno to the Black Death* (ed.) Luis Garcia Ballester *et al.* Cambridge, 1994, 237-288
3   Twigg, G. 1984 *The Black Death: a Biological Reappraisal*. Batsford, London
4   Hoyle, F. and Wickramasinghe, C. 1993 *Our Place in the Cosmos*. Phoenix, London
5   Cohn, S.K. 2002 *The Black Death Transformed: Disease and Culture in Early Renaissance Europe*. Edward Arnold, London
6   Cohn, S.K. Jr. 2002 The Black Death: End of a Paradigm. *The American Historical Review* June 2002 <http://www.historycooperative.org/journals/ahr/107.3/ah0302000703.html> (12 Jan. 2006)
7   Benedictow, O.J. 2004 The Black Death 1346-1353: The Complete History. The Boydell press, Woodbridge
8   Benedictow, O.J. 2004, 82
9   Benedictow, O.J. 2004, 58

CHAPTER 1

1   Baillie, M.G.L. 1982 *Tree-ring dating and archaeology*. Croom Helm, London
2   Rigold, S.E. 1975 Structural Aspects of Medieval Timber Bridges, *Medieval Archaeology* 19, 48-91
3   Baillie, M.G.L. 1995 *A Slice Through Time: chronology and precision dating*. Routledge, London
4   Siebenlist-Kerner, V. 1978 The Chronology, 1341-1636, for Certain Hillside Oaks from Western England and Wales, *British Archaeological Reports* (International Series) 51, 157-61
5   Morgan, R.A. 1977 Dendrochronological Dating of a Yorkshire Timber Buildin'. *Vernacular Architecture* 8, 809-14
6   Hollstein, E. 1980 *MittelEuropaische Eichenchronologie*. Phillip Von Zabern, Mainz am Rhein
7   Hollstein, E. 1980 Fig 7
8   Schmidt, B., Köhren-Jansen, H. and Freckmann, K. 1990 Kleine Hausgeschichte der Mosellandschaft, Band 1, *Dendrochronologie*. Rheinland-Verlag, Köln, 306-307
9   Kuniholm, P.I. and Striker, C.L. 1983 Dendrochronological Investigations in the Aegean and Neighbouring Regions, 1977-1982, *Journal of Field Archaeology* 10, 411-20. Kuniholm, P.I. and Striker, C.L. 1987 Dendrochronological Investigations in the Aegean and Neighbouring Regions, 1983-1986. *Journal of Field Archaeology* 14, 385-98

CHAPTER 2

1   Baillie, M.G.L. 1995 *A Slice Through Time: chronology and precision dating*. Routledge, London

2   Fletcher, J.M. 1978a Oak Chronologies; England. *British Archaeological Reports* (International Series) 51, 145-56

3   Baillie, M.G.L., Hillam, J., Briffa, K. and Brown, D.M. 1985 Re-Dating the English Art-Historical Tree-Ring Chronologies. *Nature* 315, 317-319

4   Personal communication H. Clausen, J. Pilcher and V.Hall (January 2005)

5   Briffa, K.R. *et al.* 1992

6   Briffa, K.R., Jones, P.D., Bartholin, T.S., Eckstein, D., Schweingruber, F.H. Karlen, W., Zetterberg, P. and Eronen, M. 1992 Fennoscandian summers from AD 500: Temperature changes on short and long timescales, *Climate Dynamics* 7, 111-9

CHAPTER 3

1   Suess, H.E. 1970 Bristlecone Pine Calibration of the Radiocarbon Timescale from 5200 BC to the Present, in Olsson, I.U (ed.) *Radiocarbon Variations and Absolute Chronology*. John Wiley and Sons, New York, 303-9

2   Pearson, G.W., Pilcher, J.R., Baillie, M.G.L., Corbett, D.M. and Qua, F. 1986 High-Precision 14-C Measurement of Irish Oaks to Show the Natural 14-C Variations from AD 1840 to 5210 BC, *Radiocarbon* 28, 911-34. Stuiver, M. and Becker, B. 1986 High-Precision Decadal Calibration of the Radiocarbon Time Scale, AD 1950-2500 BC. *Radiocarbon* 28, 863-91

3   Hogg, A.G., McCormac, F.G., Higham, T.F.G., Reimer, P.G., Baillie, M.G.L. and Palmer, J.G. 2002 High-precision 14C measurements of contemporaneous tree-ring dated wood from the British Isles and New Zealand. *Radiocarbon* 44, 3, 633-40

4   Baillie, M.G.L. 2002 Future of Dendrochronology with Respect to Archaeology. *Dendrochronologia* 20 (1), 67-83

5   Siegenthaler, U., Friedi, H., Loetscher, H., Moor, E., Neftel, A., Oeschger, H. and Stauffer, B. 1988 Stable-Isotope Ratios and Concentration of CO_2 in Air from Polar Ice Cores. *Annals of Glaciology* 10, 1-6

6   Siegenthaler, U. *et al.* 1988

7   Siegenthaler, U. *et al.* 1988

8   Zeigler, P. 1970 *The Black Death*. Pelican, England, 14

9   Horrox, R. 1994 *The Black Death*. Manchester University Press, 62

10   Indermülhe, A. *et al.* 1999 Holocene carbon-cycle dynamics based on CO_2 trapped in ice at Taylor Dome, Antarctica. *Nature* 398, 121-6

11   van Hoof, T.B. *et al.* 2006 Forest re-growth on medieval farmland after the Black Death pandemic – Implications for atmospheric CO_2 levels. *Palaeogeography, Palaeoclimatology, Palaeoecology* (in press)

CHAPTER 4

1   Rose, M.R., Dean, J.S. and Robinson, W.J. 1981 *The Past Climate of Arroyo Hondo, New Mexico, Reconstructed from Tree-Rings*. School of American Research Press, New Mexico

2   Rose, M.R. *et al.* 1981, x-xi

3   Rose, M.R. *et al.* 1981, xi

4   Rose, M.R. *et al.* 1981, xiv

5   Hoyle, F. and Wickramasinghe, C. 1993 *Our Place in the Cosmos*. Phoenix, London

6   Scuderi, L.A. 1993 A 2000-Year Tree-Ring Record of Annual Temperatures in the Sierra Nevada Mountains. *Science* 259, 1433-6

7   Cook, E.R. and Evans, M. 2000 Improving estimates of drought variability and extremes from centuries-long tree-ring chronologies. *PAGES* 8, 1, 10-1

8   Cleaveland, M.K. 2000 Tree-ring reconstruction of summer streamflow, Arkansas. *The Holocene* 10, 33-41

9   Hughes, M.K. and Brown, P.M. 1992 Drought Frequency in Central California since 101 BC Recorded in Giant Sequoia Tree-Rings. *Climate Dynamics* 6, 161-7

10   Robinson, W.R. and Cameron, C.M. 1991 *A directory of Tree-Ring Dated Prehistoric Sites in the American Southwest*. The University of Arizona, Tucson, Arizona

CHAPTER 5

1   Baillie, M.G.L. and Munro, M.A.R. 1988 Irish tree-rings, Santorini and volcanic dust veils. *Nature* 332, 344-6

2   Zielinski, G.A., Germani, M.S., Larsen, G., Baillie, M.G.L., Whitlow, S., Twickler, M.S. and Taylor, K. 1995 Evidence of the Eldgjá (Iceland) eruption in the GISP2 Greenland ice core: relationship to eruption processes and climatic conditions in the tenth century. *The Holocene* 5, 2, 129-40

3   Baillie, M.G.L. 1994 Dendrochronology raises questions about the nature of the AD 536 dust-veil event. *The Holocene* 4 (2), 212-17

4   Hammer, C.U., Clausen, H.B. and Dansgaard, W. 1980 Greenland Ice Sheet Evidence of Post-Glacial Volcanism and its Climatic Impact, *Nature* 288, 230-5

5   Hammer, C.U. *et al.* 1980

6   Hammer, C.U. 1984 Traces of Icelandic Eruptions in the Greenland Ice Sheet. *Jökull*, 34, 51-65

7   Zielinski, G.A., Mayewski, P.A., Meeker, L.D., Whitlow, S., Twickler, M.S., Morrison, M., Meese, D.A., Gow, A.J. and Alley, R.B. 1994 Record of volcanism since 7000 BC from the GISP2 Greenland ice core and implications for the volcano-climate system. *Science* 264: 948-952

8   Clausen, H.B., Hammer, C.U., Hvidberg, C.S., Dahl-Jensen, D. and Steffensen, J.P. 1997 A comparison of the volcanic records over the past 4000 years from the Greenland Ice Core Project and Dye 3 Greenland ice cores. *Journal of Geophysical Research* 102, No. C12, 26,707-26,723

9   Larsen L.B., Siggaard-Andersen M-L and Clausen H.B. 2002 The sixth century climatic catastrophe told by ice cores. *Abstract from the 2002 Brunel University Conference Environmental Catastrophes and Recoveries in the Holocene 29 Aug-2 Sept 2002* (available at Atlas Conferences Inc. Document #caiq-21)

10 Baillie, M.G.L. 1994; Baillie, M.G.L. 2001 The AD 540 Event. *Current Archaeology* 15, 6 (No 174), 266-9

11 Keys, D. 1999 *Catastrophe: an investigation into the origins of the modern world.* Century, London

12 Bailey, M.E., Clube, S.V.M. and Napier, W.M. 1990 *The Origin of Comets.* Pergamon Press, London.

13 Baillie, M.G.L. 1999 *Exodus to Arthur: catastrophic encounters with comets.* Batsford, London

14 McCafferty, P. and Baillie, M. 2005 *The Celtic Gods: comets in Irish mythology.* Tempus, Stroud

15 Baillie, M.G.L. 1999

16 Zielinski, G.A. *et al.* 1994

17 Baillie, M.G.L. and Brown, D.M. 2002 Oak dendrochronology: some recent archaeological developments from an Irish perspective. *Antiquity* 76, 497-505

18 Fowler, B. 2000 *Iceman.* Random House, New York

19 Peiser, B. 1997 Comets and disaster in the Bronze Age. *British Archaeology* 30, Dec 1997, 6-7; Peiser B 1998 Comparative Analysis of late Holocene Environmental and Social Upheaval: Evidence for a Global Disaster around 4000 BP. In: Peiser B.J., Palmer J. and Bailey M.E. (eds) Natural Catastrophes During Bronze Age Civilizations. *British Archaeological Reports* (International Series) 728: 117-39

20 Werner, E.T.C. 1922 *Ancient Tales and Folklore of China.* Harrap and Co. London (reprinted by Studio Editions 1995)

21 Britton, C.E. 1937 A Meteorological Chronology to AD 1450. *Geophysical Memoirs* 70, HMSO, London, 70

22 Schechner Genuth, S. 1997 *Comets, Popular Culture, and the Birth of Modern Cosmology.* Princeton University Press

23 Britton, C.E. 1937, 70

24 Birrell, A. 1993 *Chinese Mythology.* The John Hopkins University Press, 109

25 Wiener, M.H. 2003 Time Out: The Current Impasse in Bronze Age Archaeological Dating, in Foster, K.P. and Laffineur, R. (eds.) METRON: Measuring the Aegean Bronze Age [Aegaeum 24]. Liège/Austin 2003 363-99

26 Werner, E.T.C. 1922, 180-1

27 Werner, E.T.C. 1922, 205

28 Meyer, K. and Nutt, A. 1895 *The Voyage of Bran.* David Nutt, London, 1, 176

29 Wilhelm, R. 1971 *Chinese Folktales* (translated from the German by E. Osers). G. Bell and Sons, London

30 Osers, E. 1971, 125

31   Barber, E. Wayland and Barber, P.T. 2004 *When they severed earth from sky: how the human mind shapes myth*. Princeton and London

CHAPTER 6

1   Stothers, R.B. and Rampino, M.R. 1983 Volcanic Eruptions in the Mediterranean Before AD 630 From Written and Archaeological Sources. *Journal of Geophysical Research* 88, 6357-71

2   Procopius Wars 4.14.5

3   Lydas, J. On portents 9c

4   Text of John of Ephesus as recorded in the Chronicle of Michael the Syrian. 9. 296

5   Barnish, S.J.B. 1992 *The Variae of Magnus Aurelius Cassiodorus Senator*. Liverpool University Press

6   Stothers, R.B. 1984 Mystery Cloud of AD 536. *Nature* 307, 344-5

7   Low, D.M. 1960 *The Decline and Fall of the Roman Empire* (an abridgment). The Reprint Society, London

8   Giles, J.A. 1849 *Roger of Wendover's Flowers of History*. Henry G Bohn, London

9   James, E. 1999 Review of David Keys' Catastrophe. *Medieval Life* 12:3-6

10   Walford, C. 1879 *Famines of the World, Past and Present*. Burt Franklin, New York, 53

11   McCafferty, P. and Baillie, M. 2005 *The Celtic Gods: comets in Irish mythology*. Tempus, Stroud

12   Turner, S. 1820 *The History of the Anglo Saxons*. Vol. 1, 275

13   Turner, S. 1820, 284

14   Cavendish, R. 1980 King Arthur and The Grail. Paladin, Granada Publishing, London, 121

15   Bower, A. 1750 *The History of the Popes*. London

16   Hamilton, F.J. and Brooks, E.W. (eds) 1899 *The Syriac Chronicle Known as That of Zacharias of Mytilene*. Methuen and Co., London

17   Old Testament; Deuteronomy 28:18-28

18   Old Testament; Deuteronomy 29:22-3

19   Old Testament; Genesis 19:24

20   Winterbotham, M. 1978 *Gildas: The Ruin of Britain and Other Works.* Phillimore, London

21   Everett, D. 2001 Gildas and the plague: sixth-century apocalyptic and global catastrophe. *Medieval Life* 15:13-8

22   O'Donovan J. (1848) *Annals of the Kingdom of Ireland by the four masters*. Hodges and Smith, Dublin

23   Old Testament; Habakkuk 3: 5-17

24   Keys, D. 1999 *Catastrophe: an investigation into the origins of the modern world*. Century, London

25   Gibbon, E. 1832 *The history of the decline and fall of the Roman empire*. Nelson and Brown, Edinburgh

26   Robichaux, H.R. 2000 The Maya Hiatus and the AD 536 atmospheric event. British Archaeological Reports (International Series) 872:45-53

27   Baillie, M.G.L. and Brown, D.M. 2002 Oak dendrochronology: some recent archaeological developments from an Irish perspective. *Antiquity* 76, 497-505

28   Robinson, W.R. and Cameron, C.M. 1991 *A directory of Tree-Ring Dated Prehistoric Sites in the American Southwest*. The University of Arizona, Tucson, Arizona

29   Houston, M.S. 2000 Chinese climate, history, and state stability in AD 536. In Gunn, J.D. (ed.) The Years without a Summer; tracing AD 536 and its aftermath. BAR (International Series) 872, 71-7

30   Aston W.G. 1956 *Nihongi: Chronicles of Japan from the earliest times to AD 697*. George Allen and Unwin, London

31   Stephens, J. 1923 *Irish Fairy Tales*. McMillan, New York

32   Murphy, D. (ed.) 1896 *The Annals of Clonmacnoise*. Dublin University Press, 79

33   McCarthy, D. 2005 Chronological Synchronisation of the Irish Annals available at https://www.cs.tcd.ie./Dan.McCarthy/chronology/synchronisms/annals-chron.htm (fourth edition)

CHAPTER 7

1   Walford, C. 1879 *Famines of the World, Past and Present*. Burt Franklin, New York, 55

2   Krinov, E.L. 1960 *Principles of Meteoritics*. Pergamon Press, London, 120-37

3   Krinov, E.L. 1960 126-8

4   Santilli, R., Ormö, J., Rossi, A.P. and Komatsu, G. 2003 A catastrophe remembered: a meteorite

impact of the fifth century AD in the Abruzzo, Central Italy. *Antiquity* 77, 296, 313-20

5   Fehr, K.T. *et al.* 2005 A Meteorite Impact Crater Field in Eastern Bavaria: A Preliminary Report. *Meteoritics and Planetary Science* 40 (2), 187-94

6   Veski, S., Heinsalu, A., Kirsimäe, K., Poska, A. and Saarse, L. 2001 Ecological catastrophe in connection with the impact of the Kaali meteorite about 800-400 BC on the island of Saaremaa, Estonia. *Meteoritics and Planetary Science* 36, 1367-75

7   Napier, W.M., Wickramasinghe, J.T. and Wickramasinghe, N.C. 2004 Extreme albedo comets and the impact hazard. Monthly Notices of the Royal Astronomical Society 335, 191-195

8   Rigby, E., Symonds, M. and Ward-Thompson, D. 2004 A Comet Impact in AD 536? *Astronomy and Geophysics* 45, 23-6

9   Bailey, M. 1991 Per impetum maris: natural disaster and economic decline in eastern England, 1275-1350. In Campbell, B.M.S. (ed.) *Before the Black Death: studies in the 'crisis' of the early fourteenth century.* Manchester University Press, 184-208

10   Wilde, W. 1851 *The Census of Ireland for the Year 1851*, Part 5: Tables of Deaths, Vol. 1. H.M.S.O., Dublin, 361

11   Sagan, C. and Druyan, A. 1997 *Comet.* Headline, London, 20

12   Bailey, M. 1991

13   Kim, H.E. and Keith, D.H. 1979 A fourteenth-century cargo makes port at last. *National Geographic* 156, 2, 230-43

14   Zeigler, P. 1970 *The Black Death.* Pelican, England

15   Horrox, R. 1994 *The Black Death.* Manchester University Press, 129

16   Horrox, R. 1994, 129

17   Cohn, S.K. 2002 *The Black Death Transformed: Disease and Culture in Early Renaissance Europe.* Edward Arnold, London, 227

18   Cohn, S.K. 2002, 227

19   Cohn, S.K. 2002, 227-8

20   Cohn, S.K. 2002, 228

21   Cohn, S.K. 2002, 228

22   Rappenglück, M.A. *et al.* 2005 The Chiemgau impact event in the Celtic period: evidence of a crater strewnfield and of a cometary impactor containing pre-solar material. http://www.chiemgau-impact.com/

23   Bryant, E. 2001 *Tsunami: The Underrated Hazard.* Cambridge University Press, 77

24   Bryant, E. 2001, 259-260

25   Ruiz, F., *et al.* 2005 Evidence of high-energy events in the geological record: Mid-holocene evolution of the southwestern Doñana National Park (SW Spain). *Palaeogeography, Palaeoclimatology, Palaeoecology* 229, 3, 212-29

CHAPTER 8

1   Arrizabalaga, J. 1994 Facing the Black Death: perceptions and reactions of university medical practitioners. In *Practical Medicine from Salerno to the Black Death (ed.)* Luis Garcia Ballester *et al.* Cambridge, 1994, 288

2   Zeigler, P. 1970 *The Black Death.* Pelican, England, 14

3   Horrox, R. 1994 *The Black Death.* Manchester University Press, 161

4   Horrox, R. 1994, 62

5   Zeigler, P. 1970, 68

6   Horrox, R. 1994, 162

7   Horrox, R. 1994, 9

8   Cohn, S.K. 2002 *The Black Death Transformed: Disease and Culture in Early Renaissance Europe.* Edward Arnold, London, 181

9   Horrox, R. 1994, 55

10   Twigg, G. 1984 T*he Black Death: a Biological Reappraisal.* Batsford, London, 58

11   Horrox, R. 1994, 62

12   Horrox, R. 1994, 62

13   Horrox, R. 1994, 112

14   Horrox, R. 1994, 112

15   Horrox, R. 1994, 113

16   Horrox, R. 1994, 115

17   Cohn, S.K. 2002, 142

18   Horrox, R. 1994, 65

19   Cohn, S.K. 2002, 142

20   Horrox, R. 1994, 61

21   Horrox, R. 1994, 41-4

22   Horrox, R. 1994, 178

23   Hoyle, F. and Wickramasinghe, C. 1993 *Our Place in the Cosmos*. Phoenix, London, 102

24   Zeigler, P. 1970, 113

25   Hecker, J.F.C. 1834 *The Black Death in the Fourteenth Century* (trans. Babington, B.G.). Sherwood, Gilbert and Piper, London

26   Horrox, R. 1994, 82

27   Cohn, S.K. 2002, 186

28   Cantor, N.F. 2001 *In the wake of the plague: the Black Death and the world it made*. Pocket Books, London, 45

29   Arrizabalaga, J. 1994, 244

30   Note: David Austin (personal communication 9 Nov 2005) points out that the etymology remarked on by d'Agramont is a 'false etymology' and that pestilència actually means 'plague'. However looking the word up indicates that there are two commonly accepted meanings. One is plague, but the other is 'a pernicious, evil influence'

CHAPTER 9

1   Baillie, M.G.L. 2002 Future of Dendrochronology with Respect to Archaeology. *Dendrochronologia* 20 (1), 67-83

2   Baillie, M.G.L. 1979 Some Observations on Gaps in Tree-Ring Chronologies in Aspinall, A. (ed.) Proceedings of the Symposium on Archaeological Sciences (Jan 1978), University of Bradford, 19-32

3   Gunnarson, B.E., Borgmark, A. and Wastegård, S. 2003 Holocene hydrological fluctuation in Sweden inferred from dendrochronology and peat stratigraphy. *Boreas* 32 (2), 347-60

4   Steffensen, J.P. Personal communication August 2005

5   Gill, R.B. 2000 *The Great Maya Droughts*. University of New Mexico Press, Albuquerque

6   Britton, C.E. 1937 A Meteorological Chronology to AD 1450. *Geophysical Memoirs* 70, HMSO, London, 32

7   Hecker, J.F.C. 1834

8   Deaux, G. 1969 *The Black Death: 1347*. Hamish Hamilton, London

9   Tetzlaff, G., Börngen, M., Mudelsee, M. and Raabe, A. 2002 Meteorological and hydrological aspects of the1000-year flooding event of the Main River in 1342. *Wasser und Boden* 54(10), 41-9

10   Cook, E. *et al.* 1991 Climate change in Tasmania inferred from a 1089-year tree-ring chronology of Huon Pine. *Science* 253, 1266-1268

11   Naurzbaev, M.M., Vaganov, E.A., Sidorova, O.V. and Schweingruber, F.H. 2002 Summer temperatures in eastern Taimyr inferred from a 2427-year late-Holocene tree-ring chronology and earlier floating series. *The Holocene*, 12.6, 727-36

CHAPTER 10

1   Alvarez, L.W., Alvarez, W., Asaro, F. and Michel, H.V. 1980 Extraterrestrial cause for the Cretaceous-tertiary extinction. *Science* 208, 1095-108

2   Zielinski, G.A. and G.R. Mershon. 1997 Paleoenvironmental implications of the insoluble microparticle record in the GISP2 (Greenland) ice core during the rapidly changing climate of the Pleistocene-Holocene transition. *Geological Society of America Bulletin* 109:547-59.Data obtained from: The Greenland Summit Ice Cores CD-ROM. 1997. Available from the National Snow and Ice Data Center, University of Colorado at Boulder, and the World Data Center-A for Paleoclimatology, National Geophysical Data Center, Boulder, Colorado

3   Fuhrer, K., Neftel, A., Anklin, M. and Maggi, V. 1993 Continuous measurements of hydrogen

peroxide, formaldehyde, calcium and ammonium concentrations along the new GRIP ice core from Summit, Central Greenland. *Atm. Environ.* 12:1873-80; Data obtained from: The Greenland Summit Ice Cores CD-ROM. 1997. Available from the National Snow and Ice Data Center, University of Colorado at Boulder, and the World Data Center-A for Paleoclimatology, National Geophysical Data Center, Boulder, Colorado

4   Legrand, M.R., De Angelis, M., Staffelbach, T., Neftel, A. and Stauffer, B. 1992 Large perturbations of ammonium and organic acids content in the Summit-Greenland ice core. Fingerprint from forest fires? Geophysical Research Letters 19:473-5; Taylor, K.C., Mayewski, P.A., Twickler, M.S. and Whitlow, S.I. 1996 Biomass burning recorded in the GISP2 ice core: a record from eastern Canada? *The Holocene* 6, 1-6

5   Taylor, K.C. *et al.* 1996, 2

6   Lyttleton, R.A. 1953 *The Comets and their Origin.* Cambridge University Press

7   Sagan, C. and Druyan, A. 1997 *Comet.* Headline, London, 112-22

8   Wickramasinghe, C. 2001 *Cosmic Dragons: life and death on our planet.* Souvenir Press, London, 91

9   Bird, M.K., Huchtmeier, W.K. Gensheimer, P., Wilson, T.L., Janardhan, P. and Lemme, C. 1997 Radio detection of ammonia in comet Hale-Bopp. *Astron. & Astrophys.* 325, L5-L8

10   Mayewski, P.A., Lyons, W.B., Spencer, M.J., Twickler, M.S., Buck, C.F. and Whitlow, S.I. 1990 An ice core record of atmospheric response to anthropogenic sulphate and nitrate. *Nature* 346:554-6. Data obtained from: The Greenland Summit Ice Cores CD-ROM. 1997. Available from the National Snow and Ice Data Center, University of Colorado at Boulder, and the World Data Center-A for Paleoclimatology, National Geophysical Data Center, Boulder, Colorado

11   Turco, R.P., Toon, O.B., Park, C., Whitten, R.C., Pollack, J.B. and Noerdlinger, P. 1981 Tunguska Meteor Fall of 1908: effects on stratospheric ozone. *Science* 214, 19-23

12   Britton, C. E. 1937 A Meteorological Chronology to AD 1450. *Geophysical Memoirs* 70. HMSO, London, 39

13   Britton, C.E. 1937, 39

14   Sekanina, Z. and Yeomans, D.K. 1984 Close encounters and collisions of comets with the earth. *The Astronomical Journal* 89, 1:154-61

15   Walters, D. 1995 Chinese Mythology. Diamond Books, London, 187

16   Werner, E.T.C. 1922 *Ancient Tales and Folklore of China.* Harrap and Co. London (reprinted by Studio Editions 1995), 130-1

17   Werner, E.T.C. 1922, 131 and 195

18   Robinson, W.R. and Cameron, C.M. 1991

19   Stars falling at the Siege of Constantinople in 626 in a wall painting at Moldavia, N. Romania. Michael Purser Personal communication 1998

20   Baillie, M.G.L. 1999 *Exodus to Arthur: catastrophic encounters with comets.* Batsford, London

CHAPTER 11

1   Lewis, J.S. 1996 *Rain of Iron and Ice: The very real threat of comet and asteroid bombardment.* Addison-Wesley, Reading, Massachusetts

2   Lewis, J.S. 1996, 188

3   Lewis, J.S. 1996, 191

4   Jeffreys, E., Jeffreys, M. and Scott, R. 1986, The Chronicle of John Malalas, Byzantina Australiensia, Australian Assoc. *Byzantine Studies* 4, Melbourne

5   Drews, R. 1993 *The End of the Bronze Age: changes in warfare and the catastrophe ca. 1200 BC.* Princeton University Press

6   Nur, A. 1998 The End of the Bronze Age by Large Earthquakes. In: Peiser, B.J., Palmer, J. and Bailey, M.E. (eds) Natural Catastrophes During Bronze Age Civilizations. *British Archaeological Reports* (International Series) 728: 140-7

7   Drews, R. 1993

8   Drews, R. 1993

9   Mandelkehr, M.M. 1983 An Integrated Model for an Earthwide Event at 2300 BC. Part I: The Archaeological Evidence. *S.I.S. Review* 5, 77-95. Kobres, R. 1995, The Path of a Comet and Phaëton's Ride, *The World and I*, (Feb.), 394-405

CHAPTER 12

1   Wilde, W. 1851 *The Census of Ireland for the Year 1851*, Part 5: Tables of Deaths, Vol. 1. H.M.S.O., Dublin, 336

2   Kobres, R. 1995 The Path of a Comet and Phaëton's Ride, *The World and I*, (Feb.), 394–405

3   Krinov, E.L. 1960, 2

4   Mayewski, P.A., Lyons, W.B., Spencer, M.J., Twickler, M.S., Buck, C.F. and Whitlow, S.I. 1990. An ice core record of atmospheric response to anthropogenic sulphate and nitrate. *Nature* 346:554-6; Data obtained from: The Greenland Summit Ice Cores CD-ROM. 1997. Available from the National Snow and Ice Data Center, University of Colorado at Boulder, and the World Data Center-A for Paleoclimatology, National Geophysical Data Center, Boulder, Colorado

5   Mayewski, P.A. *et al.* 1990

6   Wolff, E.W., *et al.*, 2003, EPICA Dome C Core EDC96 Dielectric Profiling Data, IGBP PAGES/World Data Center for Paleoclimatology Data Contribution Series #2003-011. NOAA/NGDC Paleoclimatology Program, Boulder CO, USA.

7   Britton, C.E. 1937 A Meteorological Chronology to AD 1450. *Geophysical Memoirs* 70. HMSO, London

8   Britton, C.E. 1937, 128

CHAPTER 13

1   Xie, X., Jiang, W., Wang, H. and Feng, X. 2004 Holocene activities of the Taigu Fault Zone, Shanxi Province, and their relations with the 1303 Hongdong *M*=8 earthquake. *Acta Seismologica Sinica* 17, 3, 308-321

2   Science Museums of China http://www.kepu.ac.cn/english/quake/ruins/

3   El-Sayed, A., Romanelli, F. and Panza, G. 2000 Recent seismicity and realistic waveforms modelling to reduce the ambiguities about the 103 seismic activity in Egypt. *Techonophysics* 328, 341-57

4   Schaaf, F. 1997 *Comet of the Century: from Halley to Hale-Bopp*. Springer-Verlag, New York, 172

5   Jordan, W.C. 1996 *The Great Famine: Northern Europe in the Early 14th Century.* Princeton

CHAPTER 14

1   Zielinski, G.A., Mayewski, P.A., Meeker, L.D., Whitlow, S., Twickler, M.S., Morrison, M., Meese, D.A., Gow, A.J. and Alley, R.B. 1994 Record of volcanism since 7000 BC from the GISP2 Greenland ice core and implications for the volcano-climate system. *Science* 264: 948-52

2   Cole-Dai, J., Mosley-Thompson, E., Wight, S.P. and Thompson, L.G. 2000 A 4100-year record of explosive volcanism from an East Antarctica ice core. *Journal of Geophysical Research* 105, 24431-41

3   Britton, C.E. 1937 A Meteorological Chronology to AD 1450. *Geophysical Memoirs* 70. HMSO, London, 141

CHAPTER 15

1   Legrand, M.R., De Angelis M., Staffelbach T., Neftel, A. and Stauffer, B. 1992 Large perturbations of ammonium and organic acids content in the Summit-Greenland ice core. Fingerprint from forest fires? Geophysical Research Letters 19:473-5. Taylor, K.C., Mayewski, P.A., Twickler, M.S. and Whitlow, S.I. 1996 Biomass burning recorded in the GISP2 ice core: a record from eastern Canada? *The Holocene* 6, 1-6

2   Hughes, D.W. 2003 Early long-period comets: their discovery and flux. *Monthly Notice of the Royal Astronomical Society*, 339, 4, 1103-10

3   Hughes, D.W. 2003, 1103-110

4   Hughes, D.W. 2003, 1104

5   McCafferty, P. and Baillie, M. 2005 *The Celtic Gods: comets in Irish mythology*. Tempus, Stroud

6   McCafferty, P. and Baillie, M. 2005, 119

7   Rees, A. and Rees, B. 1961 *Celtic Heritage: Ancient tradition in Ireland and Wales*. Thames and Hudson, 222

8   Wilhelm, R. 1971 *Chinese Folktales*; (translated from the German by E. Osers). G. Bell and Sons, London, 29

9   Osers, E. 1971, 206

10   Squire, C. 2000 *The Mythology of the British Isles*. Wordsworth Editions, Hertfordshire, 158

11   MacKillop, J. 1998 *Dictionary of Celtic Mythology*. Oxford University Press, 21

12   Jones, G. and Jones, T. 1993 *The Mabinogion*. Everyman, London, 54

13   Zeigler, P. 1970 *The Black Death*. Pelican, England, 18

14   Gibbon, E. 1832 *The history of the decline and fall of the Roman empire*. Nelson and Brown, Edinburgh

15   Zeigler, P. 1970, 14

CHAPTER 16

1   Data available from the National Snow and Ice Data Center, University of Colorado at Boulder, and the World Data Center-A for Paleoclimatology, National Geophysical Data Center, Boulder, Colorado

2   Southon, J. 2002 A First Step to Reconciling the GRIP and GISP2 Ice-Core Chronologies, 0-14,500 yr B.P. *Quaternary Research* 57, 32-3

3   Zielinski, G.A., Germani, M.S., Larsen, G., Baillie, M.G.L., Whitlow, S., Twickler, M.S. and Taylor, K. 1995 Evidence of the Eldgjá (Iceland) eruption in the GISP2 Greenland ice core: relationship to eruption processes and climatic conditions in the tenth century. *The Holocene* 5, 2, 129-40

4   Bede 1990 *Ecclesiastical History of the English People*. Penguin Books, London

5   Maddicott, J.R. 1997 Sixth-tenth century AD. *Past and Present* 156, 7-54

6   Zielinski, G. *et al.* 1994; Hammer, C.U., Clausen, H.B. and Dansgaard, W. 1980 Greenland Ice Sheet Evidence of Post-Glacial Volcanism and its Climatic Impact, *Nature* 288, 230-5. Hammer, C. U. *et al.* 1980

7   Zinsser, H. 2000. *Rats, Lice and History*. Penguin, London, 120

8   Papagrigorakis, M. *et al.* 2006 DNA examination of ancient dental pulp incriminates typhoid fever as a probable cause of the Plague of Athens. *International Journal of Infectious Diseases* (in press)

9   Phillips, B. and Guidoboni, E. 1994 *Catalogue of Ancient Earthquakes in the Mediterranean Area up to the tenth Century*. Inst. Naziolale di Geofisca, 131

10   Schaaf, F. 1997 *Comet of the Century: from Halley to Hale-Bopp*. Springer-Verlag, New York, 206

11   Phillips, B. and Guidoboni, E. 1994, 131

12   Jonathan Shanklin see Jon: Shanklin-jds@ast.cam.ac.uk

CHAPTER 17

1   Zeigler, P. 1970 *The Black Death*. Pelican, England, 14

2   Zeigler, P. 1970, 64

3   Zeigler, P. 1970, 80

4   Zeigler, P. 1970, 81

5   Canadian Centre for Occupational Health and Safety (web page)

6   Pearson, G.W., Pilcher, J.R., Baillie, M.G.L., Corbett, D.M. and Qua, F. 1986 High-Precision 14-C Measurement of Irish Oaks to Show the Natural 14-C Variations from AD 1840 to 5210 BC. Radiocarbon, 28, 911-34. Stuiver, M. and Becker, B. 1986 High-Precision Decadal Calibration of the Radiocarbon Time Scale, AD 1950-2500 BC. *Radiocarbon* 28, 863-91

7   McCormac, F.G., Baillie, M.G.L., Pilcher and Kalin, R.M. 1995 Location-Dependent Differences in the 14-C Content of Wood. *Radiocarbon* 37, 2, 395-407

8   Hoyle, F. and Wickramasinghe, C. 1993 *Our Place in the Cosmos*. Phoenix, London

9   Sagan, C. and Druyan, A. 1997 *Comet*. Headline, London, 312

CHAPTER 18

1   Giles, J.A. 1849 *Roger of Wendover's Flowers of History*. Henry G Bohn, London, 30

2   De Visser, W.M.W. 1913 *The Dragon in China and Japan*. Johannes Müller, Amsterdam

3   Wilde, W. 1851 *The Census of Ireland for the Year 1851*, Part 5: Tables of Deaths, Vol. 1. H.M.S.O., Dublin, 335

4   Warner, E.A. 2003 Meteor Beliefs Project: dragons as meteors or comets in Russian folk beliefs. WGN, *The Journal of the International Meteor Organization* 31 (6), 195-8

5   Cantor, N.F. 2001 *In the wake of the plague: the Black Death and the world it made*. Pocket Books, London, 171-83

6   Cohn, S.K. 2002 *The Black Death Transformed: Disease and Culture in Early Renaissance Europe*. Edward Arnold, London, 227

7   Lewis, J.S. 1996 *Rain of Iron and Ice: The very real threat of comet and asteroid bombardment*. Addison-Wesley, Reading, Massachusetts, 170

CHAPTER 19

1   Hoyle, F. and Wickramasinghe, C. 1993 *Our Place in the Cosmos*. Phoenix, London, 102

2   Rohr, C. 2002 Lecture at Novosibirsk State University available at http://www.sbg.ac.at/ges/people/rohr/nsk2002.htm

3   Zeigler, P. 1970 *The Black Death*. Pelican, England, 14

4   Old Testament, Book of Genesis Chapter 19, 24-8

5   Barnish, S.J.B. 1992 *The Variae of Magnus Aurelius Cassiodorus Senator*. Liverpool University Press

6   Arrizabalaga, J. 1994 Facing the Black Death: perceptions and reactions of university medical practitioners. In *Practical Medicine from Salerno to the Black Death* (ed.) Luis Garcia Ballester *et al.* Cambridge, 1994, 237-88

7   Turco, R.P., Toon, O.B., Park, C., Whitten, R.C., Pollack, J.B. and Noerdlinger, P. 1981 Tunguska Meteor Fall of 1908: effects on stratospheric ozone. *Science* 214, 19-23

8   Brayley, E.W. 1835 *A Journal of The Plague Year by Daniel Defoe*. Thomas Tegg and Son, London

9   Langway, C.C. 1967 Stratigraphic Analysis of a Deep Ice Core from Greenland. Research Report 77, Cold Regions Research and Engineering Laboratory, Hanover, New Hampshire

10 Louis, G. and Santhosh Kumar, A. 2006 The Red Rain of Kerala and its Possible Extraterrestrial Origin (accepted for publication in) *Astrophysics and Space Science*

11 Muir, H. 2006 It's raining aliens. Flight of fancy, or a genuine explanation for India's red rain? *New Scientist* 4 March 2006, 34-7

12 Cappentier, E. 1962 Famines et épidémies dans l'histoire du XIVe siècle. *Ann. Econ. Soc. Civil.* 17, 1062-92

13 Duplaix, N. 1988 Fleas: The Lethal Leapers. *National Geographic* 173, 5 (May 1988), 676

14 Rasmussen, P. http://www.scholiast.org/history/blackdeath/oct1347.html

15 Horrox, R. 1994 *The Black Death*. Manchester University Press, 36

16 Horrox, R. 1994, 178

17 Horrox, R. 1994, 37

18 Horrox, R. 1994, 38

19 Ziegler, P. 1970, 16

20 Ziegler, P. 1970, 17

21 Deaux, G. 1969 *The Black Death: 1347*. Hamish Hamilton, London, 95

22 Low, D.M. 1960 T*he Decline and Fall of the Roman Empire* (an abridgment). The Reprint Society, London, 580

23 Deaux, G. 1969, 1

24 Thorndike, L. 1934 *History of Magic and Experimental Science, III*. Columbia University Press, New York, 317

POSTSCRIPT

1   Asher, D.J., Bailey, M., Emel'yanenko, V. and Napier, W. 2005 Earth in the Cosmic Shooting Gallery. *Observatory* 125, 319-22

2   Jenniskens, P. 2004 2003 EH 1 is the parent of the Quadrantids. *Astronomical Journal* 127, 3018-22

3   Jenniskens, P. 2004, 5

4   Mayewski, P.A. *et al.* 1990; Data obtained from: The Greenland Summit Ice Cores CD-ROM. 1997. Available from the National Snow and Ice Data Center, University of Colorado at Boulder, and the World Data Center-A for Paleoclimatology, National Geophysical Data Center, Boulder, Colorado

5   Schaaf, F. 1997 *Comet of the Century: from Halley to Hale-Bopp.* Springer-Verlag, New York, 341

APPENDIX 2

1   Michael A'Hearn, Personal communication, 7 December 2005

2   http://www.nasa.gov/mission_pages/deepimpact/media/deepimpact-090905.html

3   Lyttleton, R.A. 1953 *The Comets and their Origin.* Cambridge University Press, 60

4   Lyttleton, R.A. 1953, 54-5

APPENDIX 3

1   Keay, C.S.L. 1995 Continued Progress in Electrophonic Fireball Investigations. *Earth, Moon and Planets* 68, 361-8

INDEX